How Babies Sleep

How Babies Sleep

A Science-Based Guide to the First 365 Days and Nights

HELEN L. BALL

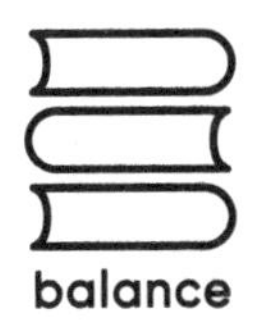

NEW YORK BOSTON

Balance
Hachette Book Group
1290 Avenue of the Americas
NewY ork, NY 10104
GCP-Balance.com
@GCPBalance

Originally published in the United Kingdom by Cornerstone Press in May 2025

First Edition: May 2025

Balance is an imprint of Grand Central Publishing. The Balance name and logo are registered trademarks of Hachette Book Group, Inc.

Library of Congress Cataloging-in-Publication Data has been applied for.

ISBNs: 9780306834639 (hardcover), 9780306834653 (ebook)

Printed in the United States of America

LSC-H

Printing 1, 2025

To Megan and Rhianna, who taught me how,
and Den, who learned with me

Contents

Introduction

Imagine the unseen nighttime world of mothers and babies. How does it look? Are they sleeping? If so, how, what on, in what space? Where are the baby and the mother you imagine? Are they together or apart? Are they alone or are other people with them? If they are not sleeping, what are they doing? Is your mental scene peaceful and calm, or are your imagined mother and baby stressed and unhappy? And where in the world are they? This last question is crucially important for our mental image of what mother–baby sleep entails, coloring our perceptions of what is and is not possible, acceptable and normal.

Let's consider three new mothers: Kristi (U.S.), Lizzie (UK) and Yuki (Japan). Their babies are three months old.

In the U.S., Kristi is anxious. She has a decent job and has been able to take 12 weeks off so far, but soon she will be returning to work. She feels fortunate she has a good employer—many U.S. mothers must return to work much sooner. She has been following U.S. guidelines to keep her baby in a crib at night, near to her bed, and has been getting up several times a night to feed her baby in a nursing chair she bought for this purpose. U.S. sleep safety guidance says she must not bed-share. Her husband takes turns to feed the baby with milk Kristi has expressed during the day, but she is worried this will not be sustainable when she is back at work. She is thinking that in the next month she must wean her baby to formula and sleep train so that she can get a good night's sleep. She must drive 40 miles to and from work every day and needs to be alert. Sleep training will involve having her baby sleep alone in another room and not responding even if they cry. She doesn't want to do this to her baby—it feels wrong not to respond—and U.S. guidance recommends keeping your baby in your room for the first year. But the sleep training books, even the "gentle" ones, aim for you to ultimately leave the baby in their own room and close the door, so she has to make a choice. She decides she'll switch to formula next week so her milk will be gone before she has to resume commuting, and once her baby is happy taking formula the sleep training process will begin. She thinks the next few weeks are likely to be rough, but she and her husband resolve to do their best to "get it over with as quickly as possible."

In the UK, Lizzie is feeling despondent. She has been diligently following the guidance of a popular baby app that recommends getting babies into a routine to support their sleep development. She times the duration of her baby's daytime naps and wake periods, trying to anticipate when her baby needs to sleep. Every evening, she follows a bedtime routine and tries to put her baby down drowsy-but-awake by 7 p.m., but she is finding this difficult. Her baby often falls asleep while feeding, so Lizzie finds she can't easily stick to the schedule or teach her baby to self-settle. She is following the guidance to keep her baby's cot at her bedside at night but her baby doesn't want to sleep there. At night when they breastfeed lying side by side in bed, Lizzie is so exhausted she sometimes falls asleep. On these occasions she finds both she and her baby sleep better than when she persists in returning her to the crib. But Lizzie is worried that by not teaching her baby to sleep independently she will develop bad habits, and that this may have a negative effect on her development in the future. Her partner says she is obsessing too much but her mom insists babies need to be in a routine, and Lizzie feels guilty that she hasn't managed this yet, even though her entire life revolves around her baby's sleep schedule and she rarely manages to get out of the house. She doesn't have to return to work until her baby is a year old, but she is dreading that the next nine months will be more of the same; she isn't enjoying being a mom.

In Japan, Yuki is feeling daunted by the responsibilities of motherhood; she is expected to integrate her baby into the family and foster strong bonds of kinship. Although Euro-American infant care ideas and sleep products have been adopted by some of her friends, like many contemporary mothers Yuki values the traditional family sleeping arrangements; she feels uncomfortable with the idea of putting her baby in a crib all alone. She remembers sleeping between her mother and father (a practice known as *kawa*) on a futon on the floor of her parents' tatami room until she was well into childhood. In their modern apartment Yuki and her husband favor Western-style furniture and have bought themselves a raised bed with a mattress rather than a futon. In the furniture store the sizes of the beds and mattresses were illustrated by how many adults and children they would accommodate sleeping side by side. They bought a bed that would accommodate themselves and two future children. Yuki keeps her baby with her in the evening and takes him to bed with her when she is tired; her husband joins them when he is ready to sleep, but nighttime care is her responsibility, and her husband never wakes. She thinks her baby sleeps well because he is touching her all night and feels secure. Yuki would like her husband to take part in more baby care, but is happy that her mother who lives in a nearby apartment building likes to help with her baby during the day, which allows Yuki the time to run errands. She is enjoying motherhood, despite the responsibility of prioritizing her son's care, planning for his future education and managing the family's finances. Unlike her own mother who gave up her work life in order to have children, Yuki plans to return to work, albeit part-time, when her son is a year old.

*

How babies sleep is both exceedingly simple and excruciatingly complex. It is simple because it is based on a few straightforward biological principles that affect all babies. It is complex because we have made it so.

Over the past century and a half, in modifying the world to better suit our needs in industrializing, industrialized and now digital-era societies, we have tried to manipulate baby sleep to fit with the rapidly changing nature of adult lives. Our ideas about sleep, and particularly baby sleep, have been influenced and shaped by the socioeconomic pressures, political philosophies, religious values, academic theories and cultural ideologies that have waxed and waned during this time. The mismatch we have created between our babies' biology and our contemporary lives has caused conflict between parents' and babies' needs—now framed as "baby sleep problems"—for which babies are often "treated" using behavioral and clinical interventions. In the cases of both Kristi and Lizzie, previously, we can see the tension created by societal pressures, causing mothers stress as they try to conform to cultural ideals; Yuki does not express direct conflict with her baby but feels the weight of her responsibility as the primary caregiver, so for her, infant care plays out in a different way.

I am both a biologist and social scientist: my background is in human biology combined with biological and cultural anthropology. This training path gave me a holistic perspective on human life and encouraged me to think outside academic silos, combining biological, behavioral and cultural perspectives. In my three decades as an academic, I have applied my knowledge and insights to parent–infant sleep. This means I view baby sleep differently than most academics who specialize in infant sleep research, most of whom have a psychology or medical background, and therefore focus on sleep primarily as a function of the brain, prioritizing cognitive development, or sleep issues as a symptom of ill-health, prioritizing pathology or avoidance of death and disease. In contrast, my research studies reflect my academic training as a biologist, primatologist (observer of primate behavior) and anthropologist. As a biologist and primatologist, I was taught to observe closely and systematically, and to ask questions and formulate hypotheses about the things I was observing. As an anthropologist, I was taught to question assumptions, understand the philosophy of science and how scientific knowledge progresses, think holistically and on a grand scale (considering evolutionary time), and critique dogma (particularly medical dogma). I emerged from my graduate and undergraduate studies with a unique set of perspectives that inform the way I understand how babies sleep, which I will share with you in this book. But first a disclaimer.

All of biology is ultimately about evolution,[1] but some proponents of applying an evolutionary perspective to aspects of human biology and behavior (such as infant development) take an approach that I consider to be ill-informed.[2] They invoke what is known as the "environment of evolutionary adaptedness," which refers to a time period (usually unspecified, but often vaguely suggestive of a Pleistocene-epoch savannah-type hunter-gatherer lifestyle or a Paleolithic-era cave-dweller lifestyle)[3] when key human traits such as tool use or language are thought to have arisen in our behavioral repertoire. In these visions of our human evolutionary past, such environments of evolutionary adaptedness are invoked as reference points to which we might look for comparisons when seeking to benchmark contemporary human activities such as diet, family composition, parenting, infant care and more; the "Paleolithic Diet" is an example of this. I would like to be clear that this book *does not* take this approach.

There is no single moment or era in our evolutionary history that has defined how human babies sleep. Indeed, there are multiple evolutionary transitions that have shaped both how babies sleep and how parents respond to how babies sleep. It is also important, when thinking about evolutionary influences on contemporary living organisms such as humans, to be aware that the process of evolution does not "design" organisms with a purpose in mind; evolutionary change proceeds by tinkering with the bodies and behaviors of existing organisms whose characteristics diverge and converge in response to their ability to survive and reproduce in different environments. Most of the species that have been produced in this way have already failed to survive (become extinct). Those that are alive today are the products of a long series of evolutionary changes that happened to result in a combination of successful characteristics that were able to overcome particular environmental challenges—not *because* that combination was designed to overcome them. As Nobel prizewinner François Jacob famously said, "evolution is a tinkerer and not an engineer."[4] Contemporary living organisms, including humans, are not elegantly designed; we have been cobbled together along a path of twists and turns that enabled the ancestral species in our lineage to survive—and as a consequence our biology comes with a lot of evolutionary baggage. We need to understand that baggage and how it affects us and our babies if we want to understand how babies sleep. It is once we understand how the key features of human parents and babies evolved—including milk production, prolonged gestation, large brains and extreme dependency—that we can understand and resolve the challenges they pose in the first year of an infant's life.

In addition to the foundations of our evolutionary biology, we have layered many cultural beliefs and practices onto our understanding of baby sleep, which vary hugely from location to location, and over time. Parents' perceptions and popular discourse in western societies have been influenced by philosophical and sociocultural trends over the past two centuries in more ways than we might realize in response to rapid social and political changes. For clarity I should explain that I am using the term "western society" as more of an ideological descriptor than a geographic one to refer to those societies that exhibit a shared set of beliefs, values, political systems and cultural norms, regardless of whether they are geographically located in the West. These concepts often encompass democracy, capitalism, individualism and human rights. In these societies industrialization, urbanization and medicalization transformed family life and baby care, setting in motion the development of numerous ideas, traditions and expectations about babies, sleep, and the role of parents that many of us are still tethered to. Our recent historical past helps explain where all the myths you've ever heard about baby sleep have come from—and the myths you've heard will depend on your cultural origins.

It is not only the public who have been influenced by specific historical and cultural perspectives on babies and baby sleep. The emerging science of baby sleep and clinical guidelines about how babies "should" sleep was influenced by the same biases and expectations. Many infant sleep research studies reflect western cultural values and lifestyles, and are what might be called "aspirational," in that they aspire to find ways to "help" babies to sleep longer, wake less often, settle more quickly, and disturb their parents less. They offer families the promise of a less sleep-deprived future. Throughout this book I hope to encourage you to consider whether studies that aim to find out how to help babies sleep more are asking the right question. The culture and history of guidance issued by "experts" for parents in western societies have shaped expectations of how "good" babies should behave and how they are created by "effective" parents while the media (both traditional and social) reinforces simplistic and outdated rules and rigid ideas. None of this is helpful for new parents in the twenty-first century, and it serves only to build anxiety and disharmony between parents and babies.

How Babies Sleep brings together the science, the anthropological context and various practical insights to explain what you need to know about your babies' sleep, your own expectations, and how to navigate the first 365 nighttimes with your baby. Often this is information no one ever tells you, or that you find out too late. Although (most) babies spend a lot of time sleeping, their sleep patterns rarely fit with adult schedules, and their sleep habits change dramatically throughout their first year—sometimes from month to month, week to week, or even day to day. The cultural expectations we have about babies' sleep habits are often unrealistic, and this makes caring for a new baby unnecessarily challenging. Understanding what babies' evolved biology has prepared them to expect, and what our cultural history and social environment lead us to think babies need, can help make sense of this paradox, and remove some of the anxiety and frustration of new parenthood.

All parenting choices are personal and different, so please accept my assurance that this book is not intended to judge any individual parents who did what they needed to do to get through the nighttimes, save their own sanity and meet their own sleep needs. It is intended to reveal how biology shapes infant sleep behavior and to challenge the cultural norms about nighttime parenting that many of us have grown up with.

Applying anthropological and evolutionary thinking to infant sleep and nighttime parenting does not produce a quick fix to make a baby sleep "better" or resolve new-parent exhaustion. But it does help explain why we might *feel* exhausted and *want* a quick way to fix our baby's sleep. It also helps in understanding when and why the search for a quick fix could be an inappropriate solution, or good for parents but not for babies. Some parents who have gone ahead with quick fix solutions (which, in reality, are often neither quick, nor solutions) may wish they had heard about all of this sooner and made different choices. Wherever you are in your parenting journey, this book will offer you a new understanding of ways to harmonize your own needs with those of your baby, to experiment to find strategies that work for you and your family, and will empower you with the confidence to reject approaches that make you uncomfortable.

1. The helplessness of baby humans

The first days with a newly born baby can be both blissful and terrifying. They are small and cute, yet fragile and utterly helpless, adorable yet unpredictable, and absolutely, completely dependent on you. You may feel confident and well prepared, or you may have no idea what you are doing or how you will keep this floppy, squirmy, squally creature alive for the next 18 days, never mind 18 years. Either way, to understand why human babies are the way they are, including coming to grips with how they sleep, we need to recognize the importance of two crucial human evolutionary traits: making milk and growing big brains.

Producing milk to feed our babies is an ancient trait. Arising 310 million years ago,[1] it is what makes us mammals, along with all other hair-wearing, milk-producing, temperature-regulating animals for whom this is a defining characteristic. Only female mammals have functioning mammary glands, and fascinatingly all of us produce milk that is unique to our species and particularly tailored to the nutritional, growth and activity needs of the babies we produce.[2] The milk that is made by human mothers has evolved to fuel the rapid and prolonged brain growth that results in the enormous and complex adult brains that make us uniquely human. Our big brain is a relatively recent trait, arising only in the past 1 million years, and is an extremely energetically expensive organ to grow and maintain.

It is usually the brain that gets all the attention, but, as milk came first in our evolutionary past, let's begin by looking at what being mammals and making milk entails, and how the kinds of milk mammals make affects the way they must care for their babies.

Three kinds of mammal babies

I first saw a platypus in real life during a visit to Australia in 2007 to speak about my research at an infant feeding conference (aptly named "Hot Milk!"). My family had joined me, with the intention of exploring the east coast of Australia after the conference. On arriving in Sydney we headed out into the sunshine to convince our brains it was daytime and to check out the neighborhood near our hotel. Here we happened across Sydney Zoo on Darling Harbour, which educates visitors about the unique wildlife that inhabits Australia. In a dark room housing a simulated creek behind a glass wall, visitors were able to observe the rare and endangered platypuses: these unusual hair-covered duck-billed creatures were swimming in the rapidly flowing water and burrowing in the creek-bed for crustaceans to eat. They were bizarre-looking, smaller than I had expected, about half the size of a domestic cat, and with a flat paddle-like tail, web-footed, a furry body and a beak like a duck. From the information displays, I learned that when Western scientists encountered the (taxidermically preserved) platypus in the eighteenth century they initially considered them a hoax, given their strange combination of features.[3]

Mammals are organized into three groups—**monotremes**, **marsupials** and **eutheria** (or **placental mammals**)—but all descended from one common ancestor, who lived some 300 million years ago. Examining the traits these three groups have in common, and how they differ, gives us a clue as to how the features that define our own group—the placental mammals—and our own species have evolved over time.

The platypus belongs to the rarest of the three kinds of mammal, the monotremes, whose babies are unusual because they hatch from eggs. Their mothers produce milk with which to feed them, even though they have no nipples, and the babies, which look like small pink beans with tiny limbs, squirm up their mother's body to lap the milk secreted from glands in her armpits. The platypus's unique characteristics provide evolutionary biologists with clues that help explain how lactation evolved.[4]

Lactation (milk production) is the defining characteristic of all types of mammal and a trait that all three groups inherited from our common ancestor. The nipple-less milk feeding of egg-laying monotremes like the platypus suggests that lactation developed before live birth (**viviparity**) in mammalian evolutionary history, and that mammary glands evolved from modified sweat glands (hence platypuses lactating from their armpits). The origin of lactation is important because the ability to feed babies with milk has been central to the evolutionary success of mammals (including humans), and the composition of human milk plays a crucial role in understanding how human babies sleep.

Marsupials, such as the more well-known Australian animals—koalas, kangaroos, wombats and wallabies—are the second type of mammal. Unlike monotremes they do not lay eggs but produce extremely undeveloped babies who, after a very short pregnancy, crawl from the birth canal to a pouch on their mother's belly. Although marsupials have nipples inside their pouch, these undeveloped, fetus-like marsupial babies (very similar in appearance to the bean-like monotreme babies that hatch from an egg) are incapable of sucking, and so permanently attach onto a nipple that supplies them with milk for the first few months of life. Marsupials fill most of the terrestrial niches in Australia but differ from "true mammals" found outside Australia in generally having much shorter gestation periods and smaller and less complex brains. The development of extended internal gestation (pregnancy) supported by an organ known as a **placenta**, which delivers oxygen and nutrients to the developing fetus, is what allowed for the evolution of the group of mammals that we belong to.

In my late teens I had a weekend and vacation job working at the local veterinary surgery, where I became familiar with the reproductive characteristics of this third group of mammals, which we call the eutheria, or placental mammals. The veterinarian I worked for operated a one-man practice covering all domestic animals (pets and farm animals). It was hugely varied and interesting, despite being messy and sometimes disgusting. I scrubbed the kennels and small animal pens, sterilized and organized surgical implements, held and soothed animals, answered the phone, assisted with surgical operations, and took samples during postmortems.

One aspect of animal life that often needs the input of a vet is reproduction, and so by the age of 18 there were few aspects of mammalian reproductive biology I hadn't observed firsthand (spaying cats was particularly fascinating). An issue I became curious about early on was why the small pet animals typically produced many more babies per pregnancy than most of the much larger farm animals. It was not until five or six years later when I was in graduate school studying comparative reproductive biology that I discovered the answer.

Professor Robert Martin, an evolutionary anthropologist and reproductive biologist, spent his forty-year career studying the sexual behaviors and reproductive strategies that are unique to placental mammals, including the types of uteri and placentas that are used to support mammal embryos and fetuses throughout gestation.[5] He describes how some mammals have a placenta that lines the inside of the whole uterus and can support multiple embryos while others have a localized disc-shaped placenta that is attached to one part of the uterus wall and typically supports a single embryo. As a consequence of the nature of the placental organ, placental mammal babies do not all develop in the same way, being born after different periods of gestation, singly or in litters, and with hugely different characteristics at birth.

The variation in types of babies produced by placental mammals means that mammal females (who are the primary caregivers in most mammalian species) need to provide different amounts and types of care to their newborns. Small-bodied placental mammals typically produce large litters of babies after a relatively short gestation (Figure 1.1). Well-known examples of these are the cats, dogs, rabbits, hamsters and guinea pigs that I encountered when working for the local vet. Individual babies of these species are almost completely helpless for several weeks after birth. Known as **altricial**, these babies are blind, deaf and hairless, with weak limbs and little ability to move. Altricial babies, like puppies and kittens, spend the first few weeks of their lives in a nest prepared by their mother, which provides warmth and safety for them and their littermates while they get on with the business of sleeping and growing.

Larger-bodied mammals tend to produce single babies after a longer gestation period supported by the thick disc-shaped placenta. These babies are well-developed at birth (Figure 1.1) and are described as **precocial**; examples include many large farm animals as well as horses, antelopes, elephants and monkeys. Precocial newborns can see, hear, call, and have sufficient strength and coordination that they are able to stand or cling soon after birth. The mother is the source of these babies' safety and warmth, and they stay close to her for several weeks or months.

While the females of placental mammal species who produce altricial babies have a **bicornuate**—or two-chambered—**uterus** lined by the placenta in which multiple small fetuses develop simultaneously, females of those species that produce precocial infants have a single-chambered or **simplex uterus** in which the two chambers have fused to create a larger space, with a thick disc-shaped placenta in one location. By producing one (and usually no more than two) babies at a time, the simplex uterus and thick disc-shaped placenta allow the mother to produce a much larger and more well-developed fetus during a prolonged pregnancy. Monkeys, apes and humans all have this simplex uterus and specialized placenta, and produce large babies (relative to their mothers' body size) that are well developed at birth. Counterintuitively, however, human babies are not as well developed at birth as we might expect based on our mammalian history, so let's

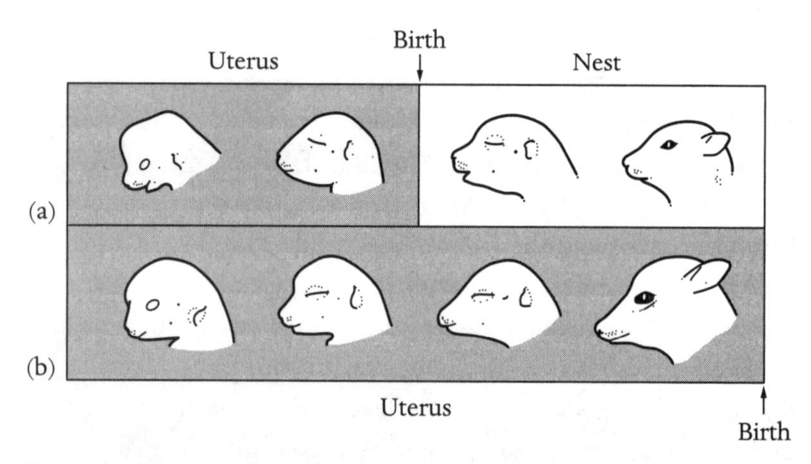

Figure 1.1 Characteristics of altricial and precocial mammal infants (from Martin, 1992)[6]

The basic distinction between altricial offspring (a) and precocial offspring (b): Altricial offspring are born after a relatively short gestation period (shading), and their eyes and ears are still sealed at birth. They typically develop for some time in a nest before emerging into the outside world. Precocial offspring are born after a relatively long gestation period, and their eyes and ears are open at birth or soon afterward; the "nest phase" of altricial neonates is thus part of uterine development in precocial mammals.

now think about how humans' evolutionary trajectory has taken a different turn.

The importance of brains and milk

Once mammal babies are born and the placenta ceases to provide the baby with nutrition, lactation is the key adaptation that allows the mother's body to serve as a buffer between the infant and fluctuations in the availability of foods that infants might consume.[7] Non-mammal babies (such as reptiles) must fend for themselves and compete for food against stronger and more competent adults, meaning many fail to survive. Mammals, therefore, have an advantage in being able to produce food for their babies during this vulnerable phase. The ways in which placental mammal mothers care for (or in evolutionary terms "invest in") their babies vary according to the type of infant they produce.

Mothers of altricial infants (rabbits, mice, cats, dogs, etc.) supply little direct care during early life other than feeding their babies once or twice per day. The nest they have constructed prior to giving birth provides their babies with safety and warmth; after birth, mothers spend most of their time foraging to both feed themselves and produce the high-fat, nutrient-dense milk that will fuel their babies as they sleep and grow. They are often said to "cache" their babies.[8] This type of mammal baby therefore finishes their gestation in the nest, and to avoid attracting the attention of predators, they are silent for the long periods when their mother is absent.

Mothers of precocial infants typically do not construct nests—their bodies provide safety and warmth for their babies, with whom they stay in close contact day and night. Born singly or in small multiples, these babies enter the world in a more neurologically advanced state.[9] Not only are their eyes and ears functional at the point of birth, but they are capable of coordinated neuromuscular control a short time after birth. Precocial infants take to their feet and follow their mothers, or cling to her body to be carried, alerting her with cries should they be separated. Precocial babies suckle often and at will when hungry. In these species, milk is often watery and low in fat but high in sugar (lactose), providing rapidly digested calories to fuel energy expenditure and growth. As babies stay with their mother as she forages, the mothers of precocial infants are often said to use a "carry/follow" infant care strategy.[10]

Humans are primates, and like other primates, we produce precocial infants.[11] We have many precocial infant characteristics: our babies are typically born singly or in pairs, with their senses well developed. They cry if separated from their mother. Human mothers[12] also produce milk that provides energy (sugar) rather than fat, and to obtain sufficient calories human babies feed frequently throughout the day and night.

But human babies are also the most neurologically undeveloped of all primates at birth,[13] lacking the muscle tone and neuromuscular coordination to either cling to their mother or run after her for months, never mind within hours of birth. So, our babies are precocial in most respects but are unusually helpless due to their lack of strength and coordination, unable to maintain close contact with their mother without help—a situation that makes human babies both unique and uniquely vulnerable.[14] Evolutionary anthropologist Karen Rosenberg observed that the helplessness of human babies in comparison with other primate species was not recognized by zoologists and anthropologists until the middle of the twentieth century, and this has since developed into a gradual understanding that our slow and prolonged childhood development is a key aspect of our biology that differentiates us from other species.[15]

The explanation for why human babies are born so helpless can be found in the key biological changes that happened during the course of human evolution, which resulted in humans having exceptionally large adult brains. Human babies' postnatal brain growth and neurological development take much longer than for other primates,[16] and so human babies are born prior to developing sufficient coordination to control their limbs and effectively cling to or follow their mothers.

As I was taught during my first undergraduate anthropology course, the two specific and defining evolutionary features of the human species are **bipedalism** (walking on two legs) and **encephalization** (massively large brains). These two features arose millions of years apart in human evolutionary history, but for several decades it was thought that bipedalism, or more specifically the way the human pelvis had evolved as a consequence of bipedalism, was what limited the duration of human pregnancy and resulted in human babies being born in a neurologically undeveloped state.[17] It was argued that getting the head of a large-brained baby through a bipedal pelvis was the key limitation on fetal brain development before birth (named the "Obstetric Dilemma" by Sherwood Washburn in 1960).[18]

Today it is debated whether the narrow birth canal of a bipedal human was indeed the key evolutionary limitation, or whether it was in fact the ability of pregnant females to sustain the energetic demands of a large fetus for longer than nine months.[19] Holly Dunsworth, an American biological anthropologist, has made a very effective case against the key premise of the Obstetric Dilemma, which is that humans would be inefficient walkers if their hips were slightly wider (allowing a little more space inside the birth canal). Instead, she argues that it is the overall body size and basal metabolic rate of human females that limits gestation length, because we are not big enough to support the expensive metabolic demands of a rapidly growing fetus for a period that exceeds the current duration of gestation.

Whichever of these mechanisms was the limiting factor, human babies are born with relatively smaller brains (about a quarter of their adult brain size) than all other primates (whose brains are about half their adult size at birth).[20] Because of this, once they are outside their mother's body, the brain of a human baby grows more rapidly and for longer than that of any other primate, only slowing down after 12 months of age.[21] This explains the human infant's curious mix of well-developed and poorly developed traits. Sight and hearing are well developed, as these are in place early in fetal development; however, control of muscular function and coordination does not develop for human babies until several months following birth, causing their prolonged period of helplessness. American anthropologist Ashley Montagu described human neonates as **exterogestates**: fetuses completing their gestation outside the uterus, while anthropologist-midwife Sheila Kitzinger termed this phenomenon the **Fourth Trimester**, indicating that human babies continued fetal-like patterns of development for several months after birth.

Although the human baby's brain grows rapidly after birth, it is not until nine or more months later that human babies are able to control their muscles, coordinate their limbs, and eventually begin to move themselves effectively and independently—first by shuffling and crawling—and eventually around the end of the first year, by standing and walking. So, by 12 months of age, when human babies are gaining control of their balance and beginning to take their first tentative steps under their own steam, they achieve the developmental stage at which other precocial mammals are born.

Now is the time when the rate of human infant brain growth finally begins to slow down, an inflection point that occurs a full year later than in other primate species (Figure 1.2).

What all of this evolutionary biology means for the sleep of babies and their parents is a central question at the heart of this book. With a firm grasp on the evolutionary history of human infancy we are able to explain many of the specific characteristics of human babies that new parents encounter on a daily basis, such as their changing sleep patterns, their need to be held and to feed often, and their distress at being left alone. The key implications are:

1. Growing a huge brain is an energetically expensive business, and a lot of babies' brain growth (such as producing new cells and creating neural connections) happens during sleep. So, we should expect human babies to sleep a lot—both to conserve energy that can be devoted to brain growth and to provide opportunity for the brain to grow. This explains why human newborns spend much of their time asleep.
2. Despite sleeping for up to twenty hours a day, newborns do not have consolidated sleep—that is, they do not sleep in very long bouts. Typically, young babies will sleep in two-to-three-hour bursts at most, waking frequently throughout the day and night. This is in part because newborns have tiny stomachs and, as we have seen, because humans are precocial mammals: our milk is low in fat and easily digested, so our babies need to feed frequently and wake regularly to do so. Many breastfed babies continue to wake and feed during the night throughout the first year, and nighttime feeding, as we shall see, is an important driver of their mothers'

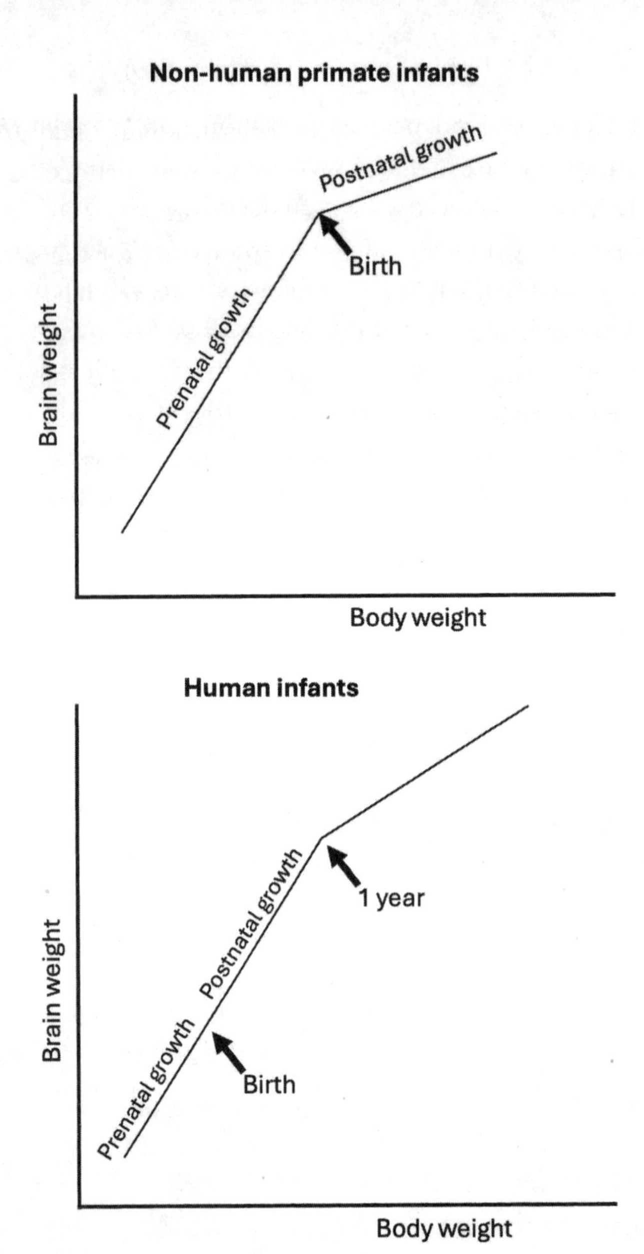

Figure 1.2 The growth trajectory of nonhuman primate and human infant brains[22]

The graph on the top shows that nonhuman primate brains grow rapidly relative to body size until birth, and then brain growth slows down. The graph on the bottom shows that human brains also grow rapidly relative to body weight before birth and continue at the fetal rate after birth. The inflection point where brain growth slows down happens at birth for other primates, but at the end of the first year for humans.

milk supply. Understanding lactation is an important component of understanding how babies sleep.

3. Related to the need to feed frequently, as per other precocial mammals, human babies are designed to be in close contact with their mothers for warmth, safety and food, day and night. While these key aspects of infant care can be outsourced to other caregivers, and even to technological innovations (blankets, cradles and feeding devices), babies are hardwired to seek out their mother's arms and breasts. Consequently, the responsibility for early infant care disproportionately falls to mothers, and in response humans have culturally adapted to prolonged and intensive infant care patterns.

Meeting human babies' needs

In spring 2015 I was invited to speak at a breastfeeding research conference in Japan. The audience comprised lactation consultants, midwives, pediatricians, and other clinicians involved in the care of mothers and babies in the post-birth period. In one of my talks I shared the results of a recently completed research study,[23] which had been novel for two reasons: first, we had used infra-red video cameras mounted at the end of hospital beds in a UK post-natal ward to observe the nighttime interactions of mothers and their babies during their first night following birth, and second, we had randomly assigned the mother and baby pairs to three different sleeping conditions. These three conditions involved: baby in a normal hospital bassinet by the bed; baby in a three-sided bassinet that attached to the mother's bed like a side-car; and baby in bed with the mother (using a mesh side rail to ensure the baby would not fall).

We were interested in how mothers responded to their babies' cues in these three locations and how this affected feed frequency. Typically in UK postnatal wards, babies are kept at their mothers' bedside—an arrangement known as "rooming-in"—but sometimes when babies are fussy and mothers are exhausted, staff will offer to take the baby away for a few hours so the mother can get some rest.[24] This practice of separating babies from their mothers following birth was common practice in UK hospitals throughout most of the twentieth century, and in many U.S. hospitals it is still the norm, continuing when babies are transferred home; the separation of babies from their mothers that began in the hospital is often perpetuated by placing babies to sleep in cribs in separate rooms from their parents. In Japan, however, mothers and babies traditionally sleep together side by side, and the idea of separating mothers and babies during the newborn period horrified the audience I was speaking to. Even though it was only one small aspect of my talk, it clearly struck a chord. At the end of my talk the podium was besieged by Japanese health professionals, women and men, imploring me to ensure that UK babies were not taken away from their mothers at night, because babies and mothers need to be together.

Indeed, multiple studies have found that many more Japanese than American babies are likely to sleep with their parents,[25] and that in Korean and Chinese families likewise parent–infant sleep contact is normal and common.[26, 27] **Ethnographic** accounts of Japanese sleeping habits clearly document the importance of parent–child **co-sleeping** for generating *anshinkan* (contentment, relief and security) for all participants.[28]

This experience highlights that, while we might reasonably expect all babies' biological needs to be similar at birth, the interpretation of their needs in different cultures, and therefore the care they receive, varies widely. In most societies with a strong Euro-American influence, the moment of birth is commonly viewed as the beginning of autonomy for a baby, who is no longer connected to the mother. In western countries, early independence is a developmental goal to be achieved rapidly by babies, particularly at night. But most of the world's mothers cannot imagine any other way to sleep their baby than by their side, and prolonged physical contact is a common theme in ethnographic reports of baby care cross-culturally, particularly during sleep.

A large study from the 1970s used ethnographic descriptions of 127 cultural groups to quantify sleeping arrangements for babies; in 79 percent of the groups included in the study, babies slept in the same room as their parents, with 44 percent sharing the same bed or sleeping surface.[29] In a similar survey of 186 nonindustrial cultures, anthropologist John Whiting found that in 67 percent, children slept in the company of others.[30] This was epitomized in a study of Mayan families, where babies commonly fell asleep in someone's arms and were taken to bed with their parents, sleeping with their mothers from birth to two or three years of age, or until the birth of their next sibling.[31] Although we might assume that where babies sleep may be similar in societies with a strong Euro-American influence, researchers have found interesting intercultural differences; Italian parents, for instance, who prefer to have babies sleep with them in their rooms, were reported to consider the American norm of putting children to bed in separate rooms to be "unkind,"[32] and argued that to separate a baby from its mother for sleep was abusive or neglectful.

Sleeping arrangements for both newborns and older babies are therefore hugely variable around the world. While our evolutionary history means we all produce babies with the same biological needs and abilities, our more recently derived cultural norms and expectations mean humans from different places and backgrounds respond to those needs and abilities in very different ways.

The lost art of cooperative baby care

During the course of my career I have had the immense pleasure of supervising a wide and varied collection of PhD students, mostly women, all interested in various aspects of infancy and/or parenthood. Several have been women returning to higher education after having families, whose personal experiences of motherhood sparked their interest in pursuing research. One of these students was Dr. Anna Cronin de Chavez, who has written about her experiences of motherhood in Guatemala, where she lived during the early lives of her two eldest sons.[33] She did her PhD research on cross-cultural variations in thermal infant care, examining how in some societies babies are considered vulnerable to cold temperatures, cool winds or moving air and so are wrapped (or "bundled") in multiple layers of garments, blankets and outer coverings for the first months of their lives; while in other societies overheating of babies is considered a far greater risk, and parents are frequently advised to not overwrap their babies, and encouraged to keep them cooler rather than warmer.[34]

As a foreigner caring for her babies in the tropics of Guatemala, Anna followed the prevailing advice from her own cultural background, dressing her babies in thin garments to keep them cool while protecting them from direct sunlight. But she was alarmed to discover whenever her husband's local relatives came to visit, or she took her babies outside of her home, she was widely chastised for not wrapping them and keeping them warm, exposing them to the potential for infections or "bad spirits" to make them unwell, or even kill them. While Anna's interest in these encounters was to better understand why there are different beliefs about thermal infant care in different cultures, one of the important things her experiences in Guatemala illustrated was the unapologetic involvement of relatives, friends and even complete strangers in ensuring she cared for her babies "properly," according to their cultural benchmarks. Even a group of teenage boys shouted at her in the street one day, she recounted, to impress upon her the importance of dressing and wrapping her baby warmly, despite the daytime temperature in Guatemala City being consistently above 25°C (77°F).

What strikes me most about Anna's experience is the sense of responsibility felt by members of the community toward the care of babies, even the babies of foreigners. Babies are considered too vulnerable and their survival too important in Guatemala for their care to be left solely in the hands of inexperienced mothers, as it often is in more affluent nations. And this sense of collective responsibility for babies is not unique to Guatemala but is shared across many different countries and cultures, played out in numerous ways.

Anthropologist Alma Gottlieb conducted fieldwork in the 1980s in West Africa among a cultural group known as the Beng, in order to understand their infant care practices.[35] She quickly realized that cooperative responsibility for babies was exceedingly important. Within Beng villages a member of every household was expected to visit a newborn baby within hours of birth; for the first two to three months after birthing, a baby's mother was looked after by her mother and other relatives while she focused on establishing breastfeeding with her newborn. On returning to everyday work, new mothers recruited the services of a *leng kuli*, or baby carrier, who would carry the baby strapped to their body using a *pagne* (large piece of cloth) when the mother needed to carry crops or tools to and from the fields, or transport cooking pots. The *leng kuli* might be a younger sister or niece (around eight to nine years old), or an older female sibling of the baby if the mother had other children. If she had no suitable relatives, another girl from the village would be invited to carry and take care of the baby nearby while their mother worked, bringing them to her when they needed to breastfeed.[36]

Shared care is widespread among foraging peoples and agriculturalists. In reporting on infant care in the well-studied Tanzanian foragers the Hadza, anthropologist Melvin Konner described how babies were always strapped to or held by someone—often the mother, but also grandmothers, great-aunts, older siblings, fathers and visitors. While the mother was the primary caretaker and babies were breastfed frequently in Hadza society, care of an infant was a communal responsibility.[37]

One consequence, then, of producing unusually helpless human babies is that caring for babies is an intensive and prolonged process, especially when the burden of care falls primarily on mothers. Anthropologists have argued that cooperation and social learning are key aspects of human evolution—and that cooperative care of babies and children was the norm for most of human evolutionary history.[38, 39] It is certainly common across a wide range of cultures, with infants in some contemporary hunter-gatherer groups spending around three-quarters of their time in the care of individuals who are not their mothers.[40]

Sharing infant caregiving with others, known as **alloparenting**, helps mothers conserve energy and stay better nourished, increasing their chances of survival and being able to reproduce again in the future. Alloparenting can be carried out by any members of a society willing to support new parents or an established family with multiple children—often such helpers are the parents' younger siblings or the babies' grandmothers, but grandfathers, fathers, and other village members take care of babies in different societies.[41] In stark contrast, in contemporary western societies, much of the historical social and cultural support available to new mothers has been lost, with detrimental effects on mothers and the care of their children, and therefore their health and well-being.[42]

In 2009 evolutionary anthropologist and leading expert on motherhood Sarah Hrdy published *Mothers and Others*, a groundbreaking examination of child-rearing across the course of human evolution. "By possibly as early as 1.8 million years ago," Hrdy writes, "hominin youngsters were being cared for and provisioned by a range of individuals in addition to their mothers." Alloparental support, she argues, transformed the selection pressures that shaped our species, allowing humans to produce and raise more than one slow-growing, late-maturing, highly dependent offspring at the same time, unlike other large primates such as gorillas, chimpanzees and orangutans who produce one baby every six to eight years. "Humans, who of all the apes produce the largest, slowest maturing, and most costly babies also breed the fastest,"[43] with hunter-gatherer women, for instance, reproducing on average every three to four years. Such short inter-birth intervals could only have been sustainable for ancestral populations if mothers had access to alloparental help. As Hrdy reminds us, "without alloparents there never would have been a human species."[44]

Useful tips

- Newborn baby humans need contact, comfort and frequent feeding. They sleep a lot but wake frequently both day and night. This is completely normal and may continue for several months.

- Don't have an expectation that your baby does not need you at night, or will cease to need you at night by three to four months. They are still developing the capabilities they need to be independent. Keep your baby close both night and day.

- If you are finding your baby's need for contact and frequent feeding difficult to cope with, seek help from others. Buy a baby sling or carrier (a well-fitting, supportive one—see Chapter 9) and ask them to wear your baby for a few hours while you get some sleep, or see if they can take care of household chores or care for older children while you and your baby nap safely together.

Key things to remember about baby humans

Our evolutionary history as lactating, placental mammals birthing unusual precocial babies who finish their fetal brain growth outside the womb has far-reaching implications. The unique suite of characteristics we have amassed over our evolutionary past has resulted in human babies being the most helpless of all primates at birth, completely dependent upon caregivers for warmth, safety and food for the entire first year of life and beyond. An important way in which our ancestors coped with the demands of this intensive caregiving was to rely on the assistance of alloparents. This was a key shift in our evolutionary history—alloparenting allowed human mothers to produce babies faster than comparable great apes.

But due to the composition of human milk, which provides energy for brain growth but does not satiate babies for long periods, feeding must be frequent and around the clock, meaning the biological expectation for mothers and babies is to be in close proximity to each other day and night, despite the benefits of alloparenting. The brunt of nighttime caregiving therefore typically falls on parents, and primarily breastfeeding mothers. In some parts of the world the importance of close proximity between mothers and babies is embedded in cultural beliefs and practices, but in many westernized settings this has been lost over the course of the last two centuries. To understand how and why this is the case, we now need to think about the huge changes that have occurred in western societies in recent history, and the impact these changes had on families and our views about babies.

2. The curious history of babies in the nighttime

Every academic year I co-teach an anthropology course called "Sex, Reproduction & Love" for second-year undergraduates. My contribution is to explore the evolutionary biology and behavior of human pregnancy, birth and the early post-birth period. I have been teaching this module in various incarnations for over thirty years. Every year, without fail, when I discuss why and how human newborns are so helpless, how their only communication tool is crying, and how they are completely dependent upon their caregivers to be able to stay alive until they are physically mobile, lightbulbs illuminate around the lecture hall as comprehension dawns. There is usually a nanosecond or two of silence as my students grasp the ramifications of human evolutionary history on infant biology and behavior, before this "aha" moment gives rise to a forest of hands shooting up in the air.

> "Why do people say you shouldn't pick up babies, or you'll spoil them?"
>
> "Why do people leave babies alone at night to 'cry it out'?"
>
> "Why do people try to get babies into a 'routine' as early as possible?"
>
> "Why do we even have cribs?"

A lively discussion follows about where the above ideas (and many others) came from, whose needs are being prioritized in contemporary societies, why this is, and how the historical landscape of politics, religion and socioeconomic development in our society has shaped cultural views and attitudes toward babies, baby care, and those who care for babies.

It is easy to see that in Western societies many cultural attitudes, assumptions and beliefs are misaligned with what we know about babies' evolved biology and abilities over their first year of life, but until we do see it, we rarely consider the consequences of this misalignment, or how it came about. For several of my previous students this discussion in the second year of their undergraduate degree has launched them toward career paths in midwifery, pediatrics, and PhD-level infant care research.

The anthropological view of babies is compelling. Once parents and health professionals learn about the evolutionary biology of human pregnancy and fetal development, the helplessness and immaturity of human babies at birth makes complete sense, our roles as parents and parent-helpers (alloparents) makes sense, and the ways in which our babies' sleep patterns and nighttime care needs change over the first year, and vary from baby to baby, also begin to make sense.

We need, therefore, to understand the social, cultural and historical context of baby care and baby sleep in Western societies in order to see the discrepancies around specific aspects of baby sleep biology that we will later delve into.

The history of Western notions about baby sleep

Accounts of family sleeping arrangements have been documented by historians of domestic life such as Peter Stearns,[1] Christina Hardyment,[2] Sasha Handley[3] and Roger Ekirch.[4] These authors discuss how several centuries ago in most Western societies communal sleeping was the norm, even within wealthy households, with all family members (and sometimes total strangers) sleeping together in the same room and beds. Throughout human history (and in many cultures still) young babies slept in close contact with their mothers at night and were strapped to her body or that of a nearby caregiver during the day. Around the world varied receptacles (e.g., baskets, cradles, coolamon,[5] cradle boards[6]) were used to allow mothers to carry and safely "store" their babies within arm's reach when engaged in occupations that were not baby-friendly. However, these devices were only used during the daytime, and babies slept at night by their mother's side. At various points throughout Western history mother–baby sleep-sharing has fallen from favor, advised against by clergy, physicians and psychologists, each group motivated by different reasons. Indeed, many aspects of infant care have changed repeatedly over time as different influences and influencers have competed to shape the parenting landscape.

What we know about infant sleep historically is patchy—but there are some tantalizing glimpses in diaries, accounts of domestic life, and physicians "advice guides" for mothers. Many of our ideas about babies, infant care and child-rearing in the Western world owe their origins to religion and industrialization. More recent (early-twentieth-century) influences can be attributed to politics and behavioral psychology. One of the most fertile sources for information on historical infant care practices and the origins of current western cultural assumptions are the advice guides written for middle-class mothers, and nannies to the upper classes, in the late nineteenth and early twentieth centuries, although it is worth remembering that these guides were idealized accounts of how babies *should* be cared for according to the writer, not practical accounts of how they *were* cared for. Nevertheless, they offer a glimpse of the infant care aspirations of the upper and middle classes.[7]

Of course, the advice manuals did not spring *de novo* from thin air. As Christina Hardyment notes, western philosophers had shaped intellectual attitudes to infants and childcare for centuries, and whether knowingly or not, many of the Victorian-era physicians writing childcare guides reflected the philosophical stances of one or more great theoretical thinkers (who often were privileged men with access to educational credentials but no direct experience of child-rearing).[8] The seventeenth- and eighteenth-century leaders of the Enlightenment, for instance, considered baby care to be relevant to their doctrines on education and the pursuit of reason. English philosopher John Locke (1632–1704) advocated a theory of mind based on nurture (that a baby's mind is a blank slate, and their experiences shape their development). Consequently, he argued that babies should be exposed to unpredictable eating times and sleeping surfaces so they might become flexible in their eating habits and be able to sleep anywhere. Meanwhile, the French philosopher Jean-Jacques Rousseau (1712–78), whose writing frequently invoked nature, encouraged mothers to leave their babies free to kick on the floor rather than confining them in swaddling clothes.[9]

In his widely read volume of 1762 titled *Emile*, Rousseau detailed how he would have educated an imaginary boy. The book included much advice on the minutiae of baby care based entirely on theory rather than practical experience; while Rousseau's five illegitimate children were cared for by a foundling hospital,[10] his dream child was innocent and "hardened" by nature, with unrestricted freedom until the age of twelve. What Hardyment terms "Rousseaumania" and his appeal to "nature" swept England in the late 1700s, and the first "infant care experts" therefore advocated that babies should be cared for by their mothers (as they believed "nature intended") rather than by nannies, wet nurses or other forms of delegated mothering (and although we now know alloparenting is a key component of human baby care, some of the practices of the Early Modern period (1500–1800), such as sending babies to live in the homes of wet nurses, were extreme). Breastfeeding "on demand" was advocated, and the use of swaddling and cradles became dramatically unfashionable. Both were derided as the tools of lazy servants and mothers to pacify their babies and keep them sleeping for extended periods during the daytime. William Cadogan (1711–1791), a British physician and writer on childcare, who, like Rousseau, championed child-rearing based on nature (informed by his study of foundlings, his own children, and comparative animal observations) and who argued strongly against the swaddling of babies to keep them passive and compliant, even advised that babies should be encouraged to stay awake all day so they would be ready to sleep at night.[11]

Religious leaders also expressed their opinions on the care of babies, with Methodist leader John Wesley (1703–1791) declaring *Emile* to be empty, silly and injudicious. Wesley and his contemporaries viewed infancy and childhood as preparation for adult life, for which morality and religious instruction were paramount. According to Hardyment, however, "sleep was not yet a moral issue."[12] During the eighteenth and nineteenth centuries, mothers and babies continued to sleep together, and this was encouraged by several writers for practical reasons such as keeping the baby warm. "The bosom of the mother is the natural pillow of her offspring," wrote Dr. Conquest in 1848. However, the mood around mothers and babies sleeping together was changing. J. H. Walsh's *Manual of Domestic Economy* encapsulated a slew of arguments against mother–baby sleep-sharing that are still heard regularly today:

> No-one of experience will hold the opinion that the mother's arms are not the natural shelter for her child, and therefore at first sight it might be supposed that it would be better for the baby to go to sleep there; and if only early infancy was to be considered

> no-one could object to it. But if allowed at that age, there is a great difficulty in breaking through the habit, and therefore it is better to begin early, at a time when no habits are formed, and when the child really is quite as comfortable in his soft little bed as on his mother or nurse's lap. It is astonishing how soon some children find out the way to obtain what they want, and as all infants instinctively crave for their mother's presence, so they will certainly prefer her lap, and will cry for it at first, in almost all cases. But if, very early after birth, that is, by the second week, they are left to go to sleep in their cots, and allowed to find out they do not get their way by crying, they at once become reconciled, and after a short time will go to bed even more readily in the cot than on the lap.[13]

By the nineteenth century, writers well recognized the need of babies for contact with their mother, but it was now deemed important to disregard their needs and show them who was boss—in other words, to deliberately ensure the care provided for babies was misaligned from their biological needs. Today's admonishment that allowing a baby to sleep in their parents' bed means they will never leave is also articulated here, together with endorsement of letting the baby cry from a young age. As we consider the "management" of infant sleep in more detail later, remember that few of the beliefs currently shared about baby sleep practices are recent, nor are they evidence based; they are cultural assumptions with roots in a particular place and time, founded on experiential anecdote, and given longevity by forceful repetition.

Take cribs, for instance. The practice of placing babies in wooden or wicker cribs or cradles at night can be traced back around five centuries in mainland Europe. Historians report that in major European cities where fertility rates were high and contraception nonexistent, mothers confessed to priests that they would overlay (smother) their babies at night to limit their family size.[14] In the 1500s, high infant mortality from infectious disease meant that half or more of all babies failed to survive to their first birthday—but while deaths due to infectious disease were considered "God's Will," deaths caused by mothers overwhelmed by more children than they could feed or care for were considered a sin. Priests were so horrified by these confessions that they petitioned the bishops to threaten women with fines and prison sentences, and it was forbidden by the Catholic Church for babies to sleep in their parents' beds so that such deaths could no longer be declared accidental. The cradles and similar devices, which had been used for centuries to hold babies during the day while their mothers worked in and around the home, were now pressed into nighttime service.

A device known as the ***arcuccio*** (little arch) was invented in Italy in the seventeenth century as a cage or frame to be placed over the baby during sleep to provide protection in the parents' bed, with cutouts on the sides providing breastfeeding access.[15] In non-Catholic Britain, the decrees of the bishops carried less weight than in other European nations; nevertheless, the *arcuccio* was mentioned as "an apparatus to prevent the overlaying of infants" in 1895 when the British Parliament, suspicious of infanticide, debated penalizing mothers whose infants died next to them in bed.

Historians have documented how sleeping arrangements and practices shifted over time due to external influences. In Early Modern England, Handley describes how relatively well-off households moved their sleeping quarters out of main living areas to the upper floor of their houses, creating more confined and safer sleeping spaces, even though communal sleeping remained the general practice.[16] Later, during the latter part of the nineteenth century, major shifts in family sleeping arrangements began to occur for working-class families. As the Industrial Revolution encouraged women into the labor market in large numbers, the patterns of working-class family life began to change. Women were recruited to work in the mills and factories that were springing up across Britain, but they could not bring their babies to the factory floor, and a mother's ability to work safely during twelve-hour shifts depended on her ability to gain sufficient sleep at night. American scholar Jill Lepore, professor of American history at Harvard, links the rise of feeding babies with milk from bottles with the "need" to make babies "sleep through the night." The first patent for a baby bottle dates to 1841, within a decade of the appearance of the first "sleep training" manuals.[17]

Big cultural shifts occurred during this period, involving reduction in deaths from infectious disease, changing ideas about desirable family size, the rise of medical "experts" on baby care, the Industrial Revolution, and a shift from a more community-focused culture to a more individualistic one, and all exerted different influences on ideas about sleep, about parenting goals, and about prioritizing the needs of adults, society and the workforce over the needs of babies. Here we see the beginnings of misalignment between mothers and babies at night.

Shifting views of babies

Perhaps due to societal pressures, Victorian-era adults appear to have been far less enthusiastic about babies and baby care than in preceding or later eras. From 1870 to 1890 "popular interest in babies waned perceptibly" in Britain.[18] Baby care was considered a chore that the rich delegated to nurses and nannies. Middle-class mothers who were expected to care for and educate their children were advised to avoid trusting their instincts and employ sound business practices in managing their children and home. A profound loss of faith in maternal abilities was reflected in the overt rejection of breastfeeding by popular infant care experts on both sides of the Atlantic.

Dr. Luther Emmett Holt, an extremely popular U.S. medical expert and member of the U.S. Child Health Committee, is considered by some to be the father of pediatrics. In *The Care and Feeding of Children* (1894) he blamed night-waking specifically on breastfeeding, promoted formula milk to increase mothers' sleep, and advocated restricting the frequency and amounts of nighttime feeds. He advised that babies should sleep separately from their parents, have regular sleep times, and that their crying should be ignored. He also suggested that it was better for babies to be fed infant formula at night, although he did not explain in what way this was "better for babies."[19] But his suggestions lent medical legitimacy to this and other opinions, and many commonly held beliefs about the treatment of babies today have their origins in the opinions of such popular Victorian-era influencers who commonly overlooked, or ignored, the biological needs of babies.

Holt's ideas spread widely in the U.S. when he wrote the U.S. Children's Bureau pamphlet *Infant Care*, which drew heavily upon his own book. The pamphlet was distributed through government agencies, which printed 5 million copies by 1930, and 34 million copies by 1955.

The separation of mothers and babies at night, and consequently the undermining of breastfeeding, was both actively promoted by and an indirect consequence of Victorian-era social and medical developments in Western countries. Acceptance of mother–baby nighttime separation may not have been achieved as easily were it not accompanied by: a) the growing popularity of feeding babies with formula preparations of cow's milk, advocated by family physicians; and b) a significant development in the medicalization of childbirth that appealed to many women terrified of pain and death during the birthing process.[20] It was in this context that Victorian physicians began administering chloroform during labor—initially for humane reasons—but soon on request. As anesthesia could only be accessed in hospitals, women increasingly chose hospital over home to be able to give birth unconsciously. Chloroform, however, was a brutal drug that left women incapacitated for several days and unable to care for their babies, who had to be cared for by nursing staff, creating the need for hospital newborn nurseries.[21] Mother–baby separation at birth began unintentionally, but quickly became standard practice. As we will see, it would take almost a century for the importance of keeping mothers and babies together immediately after birth to be recognized, and the unacknowledged misalignment between mothers and babies from the moment of birth to be identified.

The use of chloroform during birth was followed by the anesthetic-amnesiac known as **Twilight Sleep**—a combination of scopolamine and morphine. While chloroform rendered women unconscious during the birth process, Twilight Sleep provided a painless conscious birth but removed the mother both mentally and emotionally from the experience, with most users being unable to remember the birth itself. This heavy dose of narcotics and amnesiacs caused laboring women to lose control of their bodies, requiring them to be strapped to their beds to prevent injury. As intravenous barbiturates were added to this cocktail, women were again giving birth in an unconscious state, with a long process of recovery, during which caring for a baby was impossible.

Yet although hospital birth increased rapidly in the early twentieth century, hospitals were not safe birthing spaces, with **puerperal fever** reaching epic levels. It was not until almost 1940, when aseptic practices and sulfur antibiotics were introduced into clinical practice, that hospital maternal mortality rates dropped below those of home births. In the following decades hospital births increased exponentially; by 1973 99 percent of U.S. births took place in a hospital under the control of a physician, with newborns routinely separated from their mothers in a newborn nursery. Like the widespread feeding of babies with cow's-milk formula, the immediate postnatal separation of babies from their mothers was an untested and unprecedented intervention in human reproductive biology and behavior, and as we will explore, both had long-term ramifications for most of the next century.

The century of the child

In the twentieth century popular ideas around baby care shifted again. Medical and public health developments in Western Europe and the U.S. reduced infectious diseases, and Holt's influence in the U.S. extended to improvements in dairies and the hygienic transport and storage of milk. Infant mortality fell and family sizes reduced. An era of scientific child-rearing emerged in which baby care was no longer to be guided by maternal instinct, but by scientific advancements and medical experts.[22]

Feeding babies with formulated concoctions of cow's milk and other ingredients was highly regarded by physicians given its scientifically designed composition, and the ability to carefully calibrate feed frequency and volume. The most influential authority on infant feeding in Britain—Dr. Eric Pritchard, founder of the first of London's Infant Welfare Centres—noted in 1907 that regular timed feedings at well-spaced intervals were essential.[23] In a clear case of misalignment with babies' biology, he encouraged mothers to establish a three-hourly feeding schedule with no night feeds "*from the first day of life*" [author's emphasis], arguing that two-hourly feeding was old-fashioned and that cow's milk took longer for babies to digest (which was likely true given that cow's milk protein in early formula preparations was not chemically modified into smaller molecules as it is today). However, this three-hourly feeding guidance made no mention of breastfed babies, and as three hours was lengthened to four hours between feeds when plump babies became unfashionable, breastfeeding mothers (who as we will see need to feed their babies frequently to maintain milk production) struggled to meet their babies' energetic needs and ended up switching to formula.

During this period babies continued to be exiled from their mothers' beds. "The place where baby most likes to sleep is the place he must not be" announced the *Glaxo Baby Book*,[24] while ensuring babies achieved uniform amounts of sleep became the obsession of several experts. The first of the now ubiquitous "sleep tables" showing the amount of sleep "required" by children at different ages was produced by Cecil Cunnington in *Nursery Notes for Mothers* (1913). In another example of misalignment with the biological variability of human development from one child to another, it allowed for no variation between children, and blamed differences in babies' sleep habits on "feeble discipline in the nursery."[25]

By the end of World War 1, British legislation of 1918 had created centers for the education of mothers in child-rearing, where the newly established professional health visitors could inspect mothers during pregnancy, and babies from birth to the age of five. Equivalent legislation in the U.S. was passed in 1921. "Norms of infant behavior" were defined by authorities such as the American Gesell Institutes and translated into pictograms used in clinics to assess whether mothers were managing their babies appropriately. One pictogram included little clocks showing shifting sleeping patterns and periodic sleep milestones. Charts like these (based on aspirations rather than data, and clearly not on an understanding of baby biology) triggered decades of parental anxieties as arbitrary milestones for infant sleep development became designated as "normal." American parents were required to help their children sleep soundly, and the number of hours of sleep a young child was deemed to need increased steadily. The notion emerged that babies' sleep could be considered "a problem" with which parents might need assistance, creating space for self-appointed experts to jump into.[26]

From the 1920s onward two powerful voices filled this space and dominated the rhetoric of infant care: New Zealand physician Frederick Truby King and American psychologist John B. Watson. Between them they promoted a relentless and regimented approach to infant and child development that ignored individual differences between babies, families, or the contexts of their lives. Both men were gifted self-publicists, dedicated to their own theories. King's approach focused upon feeding and fresh air, Watson's on **behaviorism** and the brain. Both men's approaches were discredited in their lifetimes; however, their influence lingers uneasily in public beliefs about babies a century later.[27]

John B. Watson was the founding father of behaviorism and believed that changing the outward expression of behavior by using behavioral conditioning was the main purpose of psychological study. Babies were to be manipulated to fit the world into which they were born using the principles of stimulus and response, much as puppies were trained using punishment and reward. With complete disregard for the extreme dependency and vulnerability of human infants, Watson advised mothers to habituate their babies to strict schedules, let them cry themselves to sleep and avoid too much love and affection. In his 1930 book,

Behaviorism, he wrote, "Never, never hug and kiss them, never let them sit in your lap. If you must, kiss them once on the forehead when they say goodnight. Shake hands with them in the morning." Watson's child-rearing manual *Psychological Care of the Infant and Child* (1928) was intended to instruct parents how to create a convenient infant without any sentimentalism, and minimal affection; his ideas struck a chord with many and lurk perniciously and tenaciously in many present-day attitudes to infant sleep, such as the avoidance of rocking or cuddling to settle babies, and strictly enforced bedtimes regardless of whether babies are ready for sleep.[28]

In contrast to Watson's emphasis on training the baby's brain to be compliant, Frederick Truby King's approach focused on the body and feeding. King was a New Zealand physician who founded the Plunket Society, training nurses to visit and instruct mothers in proper infant care. Paramount among his instructions were breastfeeding (never mentioned by Watson) according to a rigid schedule five times a day with no night feeds, and "Mothercraft," which involved ensuring a baby received copious fresh air and sunshine, and the right amount of sleep, with "good habits" established from the first week after birth. Babies who were disinclined to follow this schedule were to be left to cry on their own until the next scheduled contact time. King's idealized baby, alone all day in the fresh air at the bottom of the garden, lives on in the popular notion of "the good baby" who spends most of their time asleep, with no need of interaction. King and his ideas of infant care traveled around Europe, Britain and the U.S., and for the next several decades the "Truby King Baby" became the ambition of many mothers (including mine).[29]

Babies of this era not only had regular sleep habits but also apparently "slept" for unusually large amounts of time. Infant sleep guides had babies sleeping 22 of 24 hours a day in the first month, 21 in the second, 20 in the third to fifth months, and still sleeping

18 hours in 24 at 12 months, figures which far exceed those found in current studies.[30] As we will see in later chapters, statistical averages conceal huge variations between individual babies. Some babies may sleep as much as 20 hours in 24, but others only sleep for eight or nine. For King and Watson, the parents (no longer the nannies) were now at fault if their babies slept so little. With fewer domestic staff in the homes of the wealthy, parents had to deal with their babies' sleep habits personally, adding to the need to make sure they slept long and well. Crying was regarded as an essential component of making babies sleep on schedule, and the adage of crying for "exercising the lungs" was now offered as a rationale in baby-care guidebooks.[31]

There were, of course, outspoken dissenters who did not subscribe to the well-ordered nursery or regimented child. By 1938 non-behaviorist infant care experts Anderson and Mary Aldrich had seen enough. Their *Babies Are Human Beings* became the most talked about parenting book of the year, encouraging parents to enjoy their babies, and inspiring Dr. Spock's world-famous baby manual (see page 37). The Aldriches understood the importance of aligning infant care with baby biology, arguing that infant feeding should happen as and when babies needed food rather than via a clock-driven schedule, and that babies could be allowed to sleep as much or as little as they individually needed. They also recognized baby sleep happened in a series of short bouts rather than prolonged stretches. This had been noted by researchers two years previously, but the response of the prevailing experts had been that babies had to be "taught" to sleep for the lengthy periods. While the Aldriches' perspective helped some parents, the economic and political conditions in which parents felt compelled to try to make their babies sleep for long periods continued to shape cultural attitudes toward babies and sleep.[32]

By the end of World War II, the most popular baby-care guide ever was published; Dr. Benjamin Spock's *Common Sense Book of Baby and Child Care* (1946) was reportedly outsold only by the Bible. One reason for this was the baby boom in the postwar years, when Americans reproduced at an unprecedented rate.[33] Another reason was that Spock's philosophy of baby care, like the Aldriches', challenged those of King and Watson. He encouraged parents to use their own judgment in child-rearing, to follow their instincts, and most of all to be responsive to their babies' needs and development. To many mid-twentieth-century parents, his message was a revelation.

Spock, like the Aldriches, recommended that babies should be allowed to take the sleep they needed, warning that some were unusually wakeful. He acknowledged that in non-Western societies nighttime care was frequently managed by parents and children "curling up together," which he used to justify a child being allowed to sleep with a favorite toy; soft toys for young children had emerged from the consumerism of the new century and become a widespread tool for addressing a variety of early childhood "problems," from sibling rivalry to fear of animals.[34] But the notion that babies might return to their mothers' side to sleep was still a step too far. Over the next decades advances in understanding of infant development required Spock to revise his guidance and on occasion completely change his view on certain topics (such as placing babies on their front for sleep). His guidance was regularly updated with the latest evidence, ensuring his books remained relevant and popular to the end of the millennium. By the 1980s most baby-care books acknowledged there was no fixed amount of sleep that was "required" by babies to ensure optimum development or intelligence, and that "encouraging" babies to sleep for lengthy periods at night was primarily for the benefit of weary parents, and in some cases might entail leaving the baby to cry, despite the Aldriches' admonishment that a baby should not be allowed "to lie awake screaming in the small hours."

Developments in infant development

As a teenager my favorite school subject was biology, and in my final year of high school all biology students had the opportunity to attend a two-week residential field course of their choosing on a topic related to the curriculum. Along with a handful of my classmates I attended an animal behavior field course in Wales, where we were joined by a group of boys from Bristol whose accents made us laugh. Along with learning "how" one studied animal behavior in the wild (with a heavy emphasis on ducks, and several trips to a nearby Wildfowl Trust), we also learned about the famous **ethologists** such as Konrad Lorenz and Niko Tinbergen, and how the principles they discovered about animal behavior informed later theories of bonding in mammals, including humans.

Lorenz's discovery of **imprinting**—an instinctive behavior of goslings and ducklings to latch on to and follow the first thing that they see (usually their mother, but in one famous instance Lorenz's Wellington boots), ensuring they always stay close to food and protection—was a precursor to a large body of work on mother–infant bonding and attachment in mammals. American psychologist Harry Harlow's experiments with baby monkeys in the 1950s–1960s showed that the absence of a mother or mother substitute after birth caused baby monkeys to be anxious and fearful. Baby monkeys who were raised in isolation without any form of comfort or security grew up to be neurotic and unable to form relationships with others as adults. Harlow found that providing the baby monkeys with a wooden and wire substitute "mother" covered with a piece of old towel was sufficiently comforting to give them the confidence to face fearful stimuli and explore new surroundings in a way that a bare and uncomfortable wire-and-wood model could not do, even if it provided the baby with milk. World-famous psychoanalyst Sigmund Freud had previously argued that the relationship between mother and baby was founded on food—that mothers ensure their babies' survival by the production and provision of milk, and that this was the source of the bond between them. Harlow's work showed that the bond between primate mothers and babies was not based on food, but on the feeling of safety and comfort that a mother (or mother substitute) provides for her baby. The bond between baby and mother, Harlow concluded, is vital for normal development and mental health, and forms the blueprint for all later attachments.[35]

Harlow was working in the primate research labs at Goon Park in Madison, Wisconsin, while John Bowlby, a British psychologist, was studying orphaned infants in Europe. Bowlby was commissioned by the World Health Organization to study the mental health of homeless and orphaned children at the end of World War II. These children, housed in institutions where their physical needs were met, but who were lacking emotional connection to a caregiver, suffered what Bowlby termed "maternal deprivation," which manifested in the same ways that Harlow documented for his motherless baby monkeys.

In writing his report on "Maternal Care and Mental Health," published in paperback in 1953 as the well-known book *Child Care and the Growth of Love*, Bowlby's aim was to change how institutions cared for parentless children, and to convince those in charge of such institutions that a less than perfect parent was far better for a child than no parent at all. He also recommended that parents should avoid leaving their young child in the care of grandparents or nannies while they took extended vacations (a habit of the very wealthy), and that leaving a baby to scream for hours constituted "partial deprivation." Such actions, Bowlby argued, created an "affectionless character" who had difficulties forming relationships later in life and, in turn, becoming a "good" parent. Taken literally, these ideas suggested that mothers had to devote themselves wholeheartedly to their babies to avoid dire consequences,[36] but other contemporary experts such as pediatrician Donald Winnicott reassured families that although a baby needs the presence of a reliable caregiver, that caregiver does not have to be the mother, and what a baby needs is a consistently safe and comforting person to care for them—giving rise to his famous quote that "There is no such thing as an infant…," by which he meant that wherever an infant exists there must be a caregiver, because without care there can be no infant.[37]

The work of Harlow, Bowlby, Winnicott and many others, whose research emphasized the importance to babies' emotional and psychological development of their mother or primary caregiver, is now the cornerstone of attachment theory. Their discoveries, such as the importance of comfort and physical contact, laid the foundations for responsive infant care, aligning an understanding of the helplessness of baby humans and their biological and psychological development over the first year of life with the sensitivity of their caregivers in meeting their needs. For many decades the rhetoric of Western baby care had led to babies spending much of their days and nights in isolation, meeting their mothers at scheduled intervals for feeds, and receiving little emotional and physical comfort or social interaction in between. Once proximity, contact and physical affection were revealed as being necessary for babies to thrive, it became clear that promotion of what has been called the "cult of independence" had gone too far.[38]

Over the past 50 to 60 years the push and pull of different philosophies on baby sleep has continued to cause controversy and confusion for parents, with experts advocating a wide array of approaches for dealing with disruptive baby sleep. Responsive care and attachment parenting approaches advocated by Sheila Kitzinger and William and Martha Sears became extremely popular with breastfeeding mothers while other authors devised new variants of crying-it-out. In the 1980s Penelope Leach advocated popping in for quick checks on babies who woke during the night, but being "completely boring" in an effort to avoid rewarding night-waking in any way.[39] This method was immortalized in the 1990s for U.S. parents by Richard Ferber, who promoted gradual **extinction methods** that became known as "Ferberizing." Meanwhile, in the UK many parents were following popular authors such as Gina Ford, who promoted a host of baby management techniques that the Victorians would have approved of.[40]

Anthropologists arrived late to the infant care party compared with psychologists and pediatricians, but when we arrived we vigorously challenged long-held and largely Eurocentric assumptions about infant needs and nighttime care.[41] Anthropological critiques showed that many historical theories about infant care and parenting strategies had been founded on studies of pathological or abnormal situations, and that the field of infant sleep science was very heavily influenced by western cultural beliefs and standards. Together with a handful of well-known scholars who called themselves "cross-cultural psychologists," anthropologists set about documenting how infant care practices in western settings were outliers in comparison with other world cultures. Prominent among these practices was crying. Babies in other cultures cried much less frequently and for shorter durations than Western infants, and they were never just "left to cry,"[42] although as we've seen this has as much to do with social organization and the availability of alloparents as infant care philosophy. Anthropologists provided evidence that in "traditional" societies babies are seldom left alone at all, day or night. Varied sleeping arrangements were gradually acknowledged in Western baby-care guides, including the notion of mothers and babies sleeping together, which had rarely been mentioned in popular baby books since the mid-1800s.[43]

Useful tips

- Many of the commonly heard sayings about babies and recommendations offered to new parents originate in popular philosophies of infant care from a century or more ago. They are products of a particular time and place, lacking in evidence and presenting opinion as fact, and should be recognized as such.
- Every generation (sometimes every decade) has its own influencers promoting their own viewpoints. You are not obliged to listen to any of them. Question their motives, look for the evidence underpinning their claims, and critically evaluate whether you are comfortable with their suggestions. If not, look elsewhere.
- The science of infant sleep, and the scientists who conduct infant sleep studies are influenced by the historical and cultural contexts in which they work. Recognize, therefore, that there can be bias in terms of what questions have been examined, and which people (in terms of cultural diversity, socioeconomic status, educational background, etc.) have been studied.

- Bottom line—think about who is advocating a particular approach, what their motives are, and whether their approach suits the context in which you and your baby are living.

Key things to remember about baby sleep fads and fashions

For many new parents, a baby heralds the onset of a plethora of conflicting advice about how they should parent their child—from well-meaning family and friends, and from self-appointed "experts" recommended by social media algorithms. All promise to help us find the best way to raise a child. But this historical tour through some key changes in infant care theory and practice, primarily in Britain and the U.S., illustrates how influential ideas emerge as products of particular times and places, are popularized, adopted, tweaked and then discarded, only to be recycled a few decades later. While pendulums of fads and fashions swing, some snippets of opinion unexpectedly and inexplicably capture popular attention and become embedded in folk-guidance passed down between generations. "Spoiling babies" by cuddling and comforting them, "creating bad habits" by allowing your child into your bed, and "letting them manipulate you" by responding to nighttime crying are all common examples of historical opinions that are still heard in today's cultural rhetoric.

Since the beginnings of industrialization, an issue repeatedly confronted by parents is how to cope with their babies' helplessness, lack of day–night rhythm, and need to feed frequently across the 24-hour cycle, when their own sleep needs are compressed into an eight-hour window due to the demands of the workplace, compounded by electrification of the night. During the twentieth century the popular solutions focused upon managing (or "fixing") babies' sleep patterns using tools promoted by key personalities synonymous with different "schools" of baby care. In the twenty-first century, the need of the baby for responsive nighttime care gained greater recognition, and the approach to infant sleep has begun to shift away from expecting babies to sleep in a way that best suits their parents to helping parents develop realistic expectations about babies and sleep. This offers strategies to help reduce the misalignment we discussed previously. It also explains why the issue of baby sleep is so confusing to many new parents, who feel bombarded with contradictory information. For infant sleep researchers, this is a period of transition as old doctrines are challenged and overturned. It can be helpful to remember that the paradigms governing how we understand baby sleep are contested ground.

No "one-size-fits-all" approach will be universally successful. As childcare experts over multiple generations have discovered, different approaches work for different families, and the best we can do is share strategies, support one another, and ask for support when needed. Check out the smorgasbord of approaches and guidance and select the suggestions and explanations that most appeal to you.

3. The sleep biology of babies

The first hours of a baby's life are remarkable. If left to their own devices on their mother's bare torso, newborn babies will automatically progress through a predictable sequence of behaviors known as Widström's 9 Stages, involving a birth cry, a period of relaxation, a bout of awakening, and some activity such as moving their hands and mouths, followed again by rest, some crawling or squirming up their mother's body, familiarization with the nipple by licking and touching, suckling and finally sleeping.[1] Working with Swedish researcher Ann-Marie Widström (after whom the sequence of stages are named), video-ethnographer Kajsa Brimdyr and her collaborators' incredibly detailed work documented these nine steps in a series of amazing video observations that illustrate the importance of quiet physical contact between mother and baby immediately after birth. To the untrained eye it might seem as though little is happening—which is why for decades it was trivialized and overridden by other "important" tasks such as cleaning and weighing the baby—but to those of us trained to observe closely it's clear that newborns have a built-in mission to accomplish, which is amazing to watch. If contact with their mothers is interrupted, babies may need to begin again at the first stage, increasing the chance that the newborn infant may not get through all the stages before needing to sleep, and compromising the initial opportunity to suckle at Stage 8, which in turn delays the onset of lactation in the mother's body. But if the nine steps progress without interruption, about an hour and a half after birth, and toward the end of suckling, the newborn infant, safe and relaxed on their mother's body, becomes drowsy and falls asleep.

Brimdyr's research illustrates how having a good grasp of what is happening with our babies' biology can help us work out how we can support and work with these biological processes rather than unwittingly and unhelpfully fighting against them. Such research has helped change delivery room practices immediately after birth, such as cleaning, weighing and dressing babies, separating them from their mothers, and placing them on their own in a cold crib, all of which interfere with the unfolding of normal post-birth biology and behavior.

Many key aspects of parent–baby biology, such as lactation and touch, interact with the biology and behavior of baby sleep, as the primary needs of babies for sleep, food and contact are inextricably intertwined. Insights about how this all works and affects our babies' sleep can help us think through how we might respond to our babies' cues and meet their needs in the first few days and months of life, how our baby's capabilities might fit with our personal parenting goals and values, and help us adjust our expectations to be realistic.

As we have seen, "normal baby sleep" has been framed in many different ways, and historical views have changed dramatically from one decade to the next.

Still today, there are stark contradictions and conflicting notions about what we should expect of our babies, and of ourselves as parents. When we have a particular expectation in mind that our baby is not meeting, it can lead to distress, anxiety, and a concern that either we might be doing something wrong or that something is wrong with our baby. Knowing how the biology of babies and the biology of sleep work can help you better understand how your baby *really* sleeps, what things influence their sleep patterns, and how your baby might vary from another.

What is sleep and why do we do it?

While we intuitively understand what happens when we sleep—after all, we all do it, all the time—for scientists, describing what sleep entails is not easy, as being asleep (like being awake) is a dynamic process rather than a simple state. We are not conscious, but we are not fully unconscious either as our apparent unconsciousness is quickly reversible (unlike, for instance, being unconscious in a coma, or under the influence of anesthesia).

Understanding the function of sleep is not particularly straightforward either, and the explanations you hear may depend, unsurprisingly, on the academic backgrounds of the experts you ask. Several well-known explanations relate the function of sleep to: a) restoration and recovery; b) energy conservation; and c) memory and cognitive function.

Biologists emphasize the role of sleep in the repair, restoration and recovery of the brain and body on a physiological and cellular level—our bodies need downtime in order to repair themselves and restore equilibrium. This can be observed in our increased need for sleep when our bodies are fighting infection or recovering from injury, and the well-known relationship between growth and sleep. The repair and restore function of sleep may also extend to removing toxic chemicals from the brain that build up during wakefulness, such as beta-amyloids, which are implicated in diseases such as Alzheimer's.

Behavioral ecologists, on the other hand, emphasize the energy conservation function of sleep, pointing out that sleeping for a substantial period each day is a strategy for reducing an organism's energy consumption and ensuring animals (including humans) do not expend more calories than they can acquire and consume. For babies' bodies the energy-conservation function of sleep may be rather important as infancy is a phase when energy is invested in rapid growth, as well as repair and restoration. This provides some explanation for why we need so much more sleep in early life than we do as we age, when our energetic demands reduce due to lack of growth and lower activity levels. However, for species with brains as big as ours, sleeping still uses energy, so the amount saved is not huge.

Psychologists argue that we sleep to allow the brain the opportunity to process and codify the information acquired during waking hours, and it has been demonstrated in multiple experiments with adults and children that sleep improves learning and cognitive function. These processes are supported by neural plasticity, whereby the brain forms and reforms neural connections and networks during sleep. As every new experience is a learning opportunity, human babies' brains are creating neural pathways at a phenomenal rate throughout the first year of life, hence the rapid increase in brain size between birth and a child's first birthday, at which point brain growth eventually begins to slow down (Figure 1.2).

None of these explanations for the role of sleep are mutually exclusive, and more recent untested theories also exist, such as the role of sleep in emotional regulation, so it is likely that sleep serves several functions, and perhaps has different functions for different animals, or at different phases of the lifespan.

Sleep, then, is not just the absence of waking—during sleep our brains do not simply "switch off"; in fact, during some periods of sleep our brains are just as active as when we are awake.

Sleep architecture

The activity of the sleeping brain can be measured via **polysomnography**, a process that uses electrodes positioned on the outside of the skull to measure the electrical impulses traveling through the brain (**electroencephalography** or **EEG**). These electrical impulses—or "brain waves," as they are more commonly known—have different amplitudes (signal strength) that are used to distinguish between different stages of sleep, ranging from the **REM (Rapid Eye Movement)** stage to deep **non-REM** (or NREM) sleep. While our brains are busy processing information when we are awake and when we are in REM sleep, non-REM sleep is the phase when the brain is relatively quiet and sleep is restful and restorative. If we were to look at an EEG trace of your brain's activity now, while you are reading, you would see a squiggly line on a computer screen that showed erratic and fast but small oscillations, like densely packed but irregular teeth on a saw, which is also how brain waves appear during REM sleep, although perhaps a bit less densely packed. In contrast, when you are in deep sleep, the waves would be much deeper, even more irregular in shape, and spaced farther apart, looking more like jagged rocks. During REM sleep our eyes move quickly underneath our closed eyelids and our bodies are still and limp, while in non-REM sleep there are no eye movements, and our muscles are functional, allowing us to move our limbs and change body position.

Sleep, then, has a cyclic or rhythmic organization that alternates between REM and non-REM. These alternating patterns, known as sleep cycles or **ultradian rhythms**, are often depicted using a chart called a **hypnogram** (literally a sleep graph; Figure 3.1), which shows how they change throughout a sleep period (typically across a night).

As this hypnogram shows, when adults fall asleep we pass quickly through the sleep stages from awake to deep sleep (NREM3), spend 30 to 60 minutes in deep sleep, and then begin to move back through the sleep stages to REM sleep. Overall, a full sleep cycle lasts for about 90 minutes, and then the pattern is repeated. As a sleep period progresses, we spend a smaller proportion of time in deep sleep and more time in REM sleep during each successive cycle. Toward the end of our sleep period most of our sleep occurs in the lighter stages, with some complete arousals (periods of waking) in the second part of the night. The sequence of the different types of activity our brains are engaged in during sleep, and the duration of each type, is termed our **sleep architecture**, which varies in its key characteristics across our lifespan.

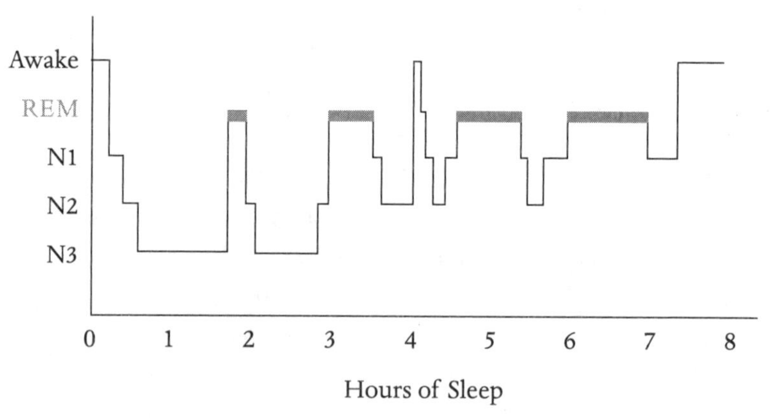

Figure 3.1 Adult hypnogram illustrating sleep cycles and preponderance of deep sleep at the beginning of the night, and REM sleep toward the end of the night

What's different about baby sleep?

We know from evolutionary biology that human babies spend their first months of life finishing gestation outside the womb, their brains growing and developing rapidly (in what is termed the fourth trimester). Although babies generally sleep a lot during this period, they sleep very differently from their parents in both visible and invisible ways. Newborn babies spend much more time asleep than adults, as their brains process information and grow. They don't sleep all night, and they don't sleep only at night as they have no body clock (**circadian rhythm**). They have shorter sleep cycles and spend much more time in what is known as **Active sleep**, which is the infant equivalent of REM sleep. Over time babies' sleep biology matures and begins to more closely resemble adult sleep, with longer sleep cycles, and deep sleep consolidated in the first half of the night, but the development of this is apparent in bursts and starts rather than as a gradual and continuous process.

As far as we know, during gestation, babies spend most (up to 95%) of their time asleep,[2] and fetal sleep, it seems, can be differentiated into Active and **Quiet sleep** by around 23 weeks gestation.[3] Researchers have assessed that up to 80 percent of fetal sleep time is spent in Active sleep during the last trimester, presumably because this is the sleep stage in which the brain is actively growing—fetal brains grow rapidly, creating masses of neural connections (synaptogenesis), in the final weeks before birth. This means that a premature baby born at 30 weeks will spend much more time in Active sleep than a full-term newborn, and their sleep will be more fragmented with shorter sleep cycles and more frequent arousals while synaptogenesis occurs. Premature infants may have difficulty transitioning smoothly from one sleep cycle to another due to the immaturity of their central nervous system. Over time, aspects of sleep development such as circadian development and nighttime **sleep consolidation** will be correspondingly delayed. For premature babies in neonatal care units, therefore, it is important to protect sleep so that brain development is not disrupted.[4] This appears to be best achieved by the use of **skin-to-skin contact** (also known as Kangaroo Mother Care).[5]

For full-term babies, in the first few months after birth, sleep time is almost equally split between Active sleep and Quiet sleep—meaning that for 50 percent of your baby's sleep time (up to 10 hours a day), their brains are actively processing new information that was acquired while they were awake, the key function of Active sleep. As babies develop and their brains mature, they begin to sleep for fewer hours and spend a smaller proportion of their sleep time in Active (REM) sleep. By adulthood we spend less than 20 percent of our total sleep time in REM sleep (Figure 3.2), and total sleep time within 24 hours diminishes as we age.

Over the first year of postnatal life, sleep is the primary activity of the developing brain, and babies' brains are incredibly active

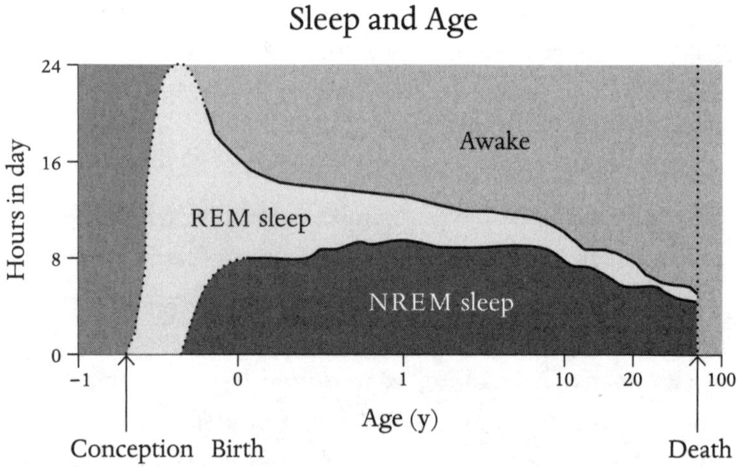

Sleep and Age

Figure 3.2 Active/REM sleep by age

At birth, the newborn infant spends approximately 50% of sleep time in REM sleep, but by age 6 years, this time is decreased to the normal adult pattern of 25%.

during sleep, much more so than in adulthood—in fact the sleeping brain is more active during infancy than at any other period of our lives. You can easily see this if you compare the hypnogram below (Figure 3.3) of a sleeping newborn with that of an adult in Figure 3.1. A baby's hypnogram is a lot messier than an adult's, with many spikes of wakefulness.

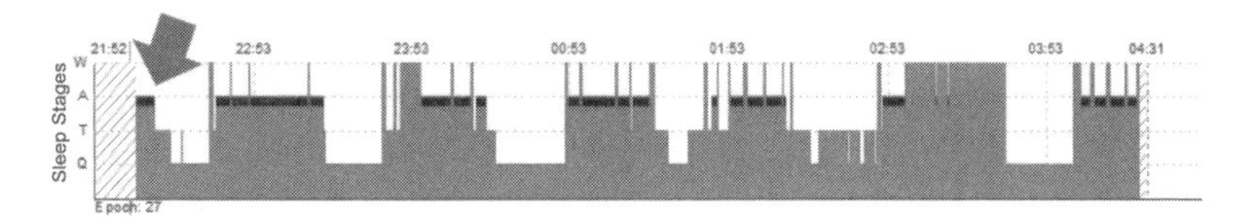

Figure 3.3. Infant hypnogram (0–2 months of age) illustrating sleep cycles, preponderance of active sleep across the sleep period, and frequent brief arousals, with full awakenings every 2–3 hours.[6]

Sleep stages are more difficult to identify using EEG in infants than in adults, as babies' brains and brain waves are not yet mature, so infant sleep stages are classified in four generic categories encompassing Wake, Active sleep, Transient or Indeterminate sleep, and Quiet sleep.

As we have discussed, Active sleep is the infant equivalent of REM sleep in adults. If you watch a newborn during Active sleep, you will often see them sucking, twitching, frowning, breathing irregularly and moving their limbs—so much so that they might be mistaken for being awake. The typical muscle paralysis that makes us lie motionless during REM sleep does not develop until the middle of a baby's first year, when the nervous system has sufficiently matured. It is at this time that adult forms of REM and non-REM sleep gradually begin to appear, and you will begin to see your baby become less active and twitchy when they are asleep. By six months or so REM stillness (muscle paralysis) will appear, and when you pick your sleeping baby up their limbs and body will be floppy. In contrast, when they are in Quiet sleep babies will breathe rhythmically and make large limb and whole body movements; their body is relaxed, and they are sleeping most deeply. Transient or indeterminate sleep cannot be clearly defined as either Active or Quiet sleep using polysomnography, but it is a stage babies pass through—and sometimes stay in for a while—as they progress between sleep cycles.

As the infant hypnogram (Figure 3.3) shows, when young babies fall asleep they do not fall quickly into deeper sleep as adults do, but linger for a while in Active sleep (see arrow) before progressing through Transient to Quiet sleep. This process takes around 20–30 minutes, during which babies are easily rousable. Babies will follow this process for the first three to six months of life, and their sleep cycles are 45–60 minutes long.

Newborns spontaneously wake between (not during) sleep cycles, sometimes after just one, but often young babies will wake after every second or third sleep cycle during the first couple of months after birth. As their brain matures, some babies will begin to smoothly transition into the next cycle, perhaps sleeping for four or five sleep cycles in a row before waking at night, a phenomenon known as sleep consolidation. We will discuss the research around sleep consolidation in Chapter 4, however for now it is useful to know that although you may read a lot about the importance of babies "settling" or developing sleep consolidation at around three to four months, only about a third of babies do this while the majority continue to wake at the end of every couple of sleep cycles. Furthermore, those who *do* begin to sleep for longer stretches in their third month don't necessarily retain this sleep pattern in their fourth month as developmental changes occurring around this time often trigger babies to resume night-waking. While some authors refer to this phenomenon as a "sleep regression," this has no biological basis; it is more helpful to frame these periods of sleep disruption as normal consequences of periods of intense neurological development linked with the acquisition of new skills (see Chapter 4).

Useful tip

If, in the first few months, your baby falls asleep on you, and you intend to transfer them to a crib or other sleep surface, do not move them too soon! Observe their movements and breathing to identify when they are in deep sleep before trying to move them; they are less likely to wake up during the change of location once they are in this stage, so long as they are handled gently.

Understanding sleep architecture helps us to make sense of the cyclical rhythms of sleep cycles and sleep stages that are triggered whenever we or our babies fall asleep. But there are other biological rhythms that influence when we might sleep and wake up. These are known as the **biological sleep regulators**, commonly referred to as the **circadian cycle** or body clock, and **sleep pressure**.

Body clocks and sleep pressure

So far we have considered what happens *during* sleep. But this doesn't tell us anything about the process of how, when and why babies fall asleep in the first place.

The timing of sleep—in babies as in adults—is controlled by two biological systems that regulate when we sleep and how long we sleep for. One of these is the circadian clock (also known as Process C), which is driven by an area of the brain embedded within the hypothalamus—a structure deep within your brain—called the **Suprachiasmatic Nucleus** (SCN). The SCN synchronizes our bodies with environmental cues (or **zeitgebers**), such as daylight, activity and noise. It also serves as the master clock for biological rhythms in mammals, and the activity of all animals is linked in some way to cues from the external environment: male birds are triggered to sing in the spring by increasing day length;[7] horseshoe crabs on the East Coast of America retreat up the coastline in synchrony with the rising tide on their native beaches, even if they are moved hundreds of miles away from that location;[8] and diurnal mammals (i.e., those awake during the daytime) are nudged toward sleepiness by the gradual onset of darkness.[9]

During gestation, the developing baby has no independent circadian rhythm; their daily biological cycles (such as the cyclical release of hormones) are controlled by their mother's body clock. After birth a newborn has not yet developed their own day–night rhythm and will sleep and wake with equal frequency throughout the daytime and the nighttime. Babies' circadian patterns mature over the first year of life, with the first signs of circadian functions beginning to appear around three to four months of age.[10] Although you can't observe this, a four-month-old baby will have a measurable cortisol peak in the morning and melatonin peak in the evening, and they will experience a reduction in body temperature an hour or so after sleep onset. What you may notice is them starting to spend more time asleep during nighttime hours, and more time awake during daylight, even if their sleep is not yet consolidated and they still wake frequently. As babies' circadian clocks begin to mature, their development can be supported by regular exposure to daylight (by being taken outside) early in the day, so the daylight begins to entrain the SCN.[11] Although it is often advised that babies should take daytime sleep in dark and silent rooms in order to encourage prolonged and deep sleep (and to "teach" babies that darkness = sleep time), this does not support, and in fact disrupts, the developing circadian rhythm.

Useful tip

To help a baby's day–night cycle develop, and to support sleep consolidation at night over the first year, keep your baby in the daylight during daytime sleep. Daylight, noise and activity are all helpful circadian cues, and their effects are suppressed by moving babies into quiet, darkened rooms for sleep during the day.

While many people are aware of circadian rhythms and their role in modulating sleep and wake cycles, the other key biological sleep regulator that drives our sleep timing, known as sleep pressure, is less familiar, and its role in infant sleep is typically unknown to parents. My research collaborator Dr. Pam Douglas, who founded the Possums Clinic for Mothers & Babies in Brisbane, Australia, and who now runs the NDC Institute: Home of Possums, explains sleep pressure by asking parents to imagine that they have arrived home from a busy day at work. They sit down on the sofa at around 7 p.m. and, as they begin to relax, they think to themselves: "If I just close my eyes now, I would be asleep in no time." This is because their sleep pressure is rising and their body feels the urge to take the edge off it with a nap. But they know that if they do fall asleep there on the couch at 7 p.m., they'll wake in an hour or two and then won't be able to fall back to sleep at their normal bedtime. This is because once they've had a nap, their sleep pressure has reduced, and they will no longer feel the urge to sleep again so soon. However, if at 7 p.m. they get up from the couch and make their dinner, watch some TV, and otherwise make themselves stay awake for a few more hours, their sleep pressure will keep rising and so by the time they do go to bed, their sleep pressure will be so high that they are likely to be asleep within moments of putting their head on the pillow. When sleep pressure is high and the conditions for sleep are right, sleep happens easily.

Sleep pressure (technically named the **sleep–wake homeostat** or Process S) is the progressively inevitable urge to sleep that we experience the longer we stay awake, and that reduces when we sleep. The longer we are awake the more sleep pressure rises. Typically, sleep happens most easily for adults when sleep pressure has built up over a 14–16-hour period. If we were to try to force ourselves to stay awake over a long enough period, eventually we would fall asleep even though we were trying not to, and if prevented from doing so we would begin to hallucinate and lose our mental stability.[12]

A particularly vivid demonstration of this took place in 2005 when an American documentary followed a group of people in Texas who were competing to win a brand-new truck.[13] The winner would be the person who could remain touching the truck for the longest period. Sleep deprivation and the relentless build-up of sleep pressure was the key challenge to be endured in order to win. After several days, one of the contestants, deranged by sleep deprivation, broke into a nearby store during one of the toilet breaks, took a shotgun from the sporting goods section, and killed himself. A lawsuit brought by his widow against the dealership that ran the competition argued that the stress and sleep deprivation experienced by her husband and other contestants was like "brainwashing," and that the contestants "temporarily lost their sanity."[14] Attempting to override sleep pressure for prolonged periods is extreme and ill-advised.

The sensation we experience as sleep pressure is caused by the buildup of chemicals (known as adenosines) in the brain. Adenosines are proteins with a wide range of functions in mammalian biology, which are present in the brains of newborn babies from birth, driving their need to sleep after relatively short periods of time awake. These proteins accumulate while we are awake and are removed from our brains while we sleep. If we delay sleep, the buildup of adenosines cannot go on unchecked. At some point, eventually, we must sleep, and for babies this happens much more quickly than for adults. However, we can only fall asleep when our bodies are relaxed and our brains are ready to switch off. We can override sleep pressure for a short while (due to stimulants, pain, anxiety, fear), but as these wear off sleep pressure will again take over. When people are suffering with chronic stress or grief that prevents them from calming themselves sufficiently to be able to fall asleep, they may be prescribed tranquilizers (relaxants) to help them unwind enough for sleep pressure to initiate sleep.

For babies, then, sleep pressure builds up much more quickly than for adults (Figure 3.4). In this diagram, the adult is able to sustain a long period of wakefulness from morning until evening before sleep pressure is experienced, while during the same period the baby's sleep pressure accumulates to the point where they must sleep three times. In this depiction the baby only sleeps for long enough to take the immediate edge off their sleep pressure and keep it climbing toward nighttime, which facilitates sleeping for longer stretches at night once babies are past the first few months of age. Young babies often fall asleep after being awake for an hour or two, but as children get older sleep pressure builds more slowly. It takes two to three years until a child can consistently stay awake all day.

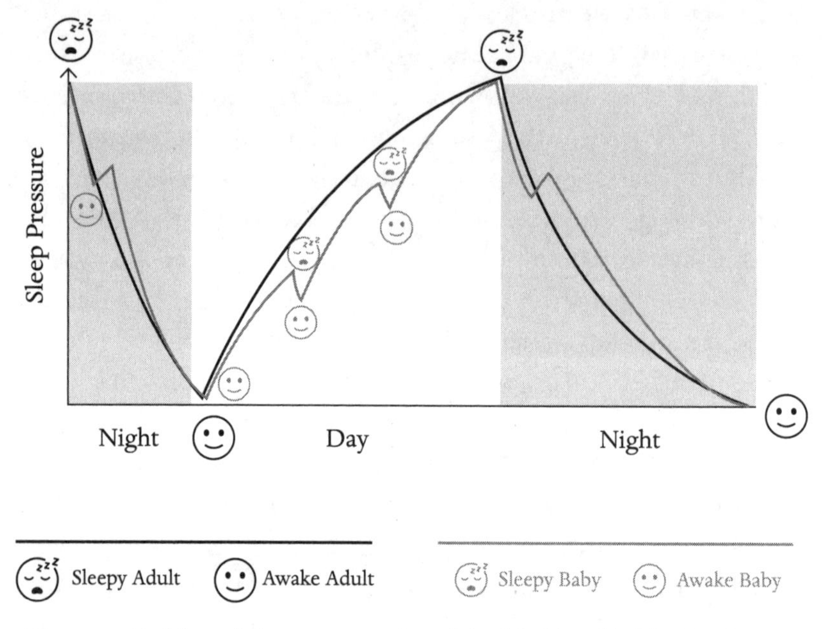

Figure 3.4 Buildup of sleep pressure for adults (black) and babies (gray)

In the newborn period some babies will spend almost all their time asleep while others are able to sustain wakefulness for 45 minutes to an hour at a time; by two to three months of age babies are generally able to stay awake for between one and two hours before sleep pressure has sufficiently built up that they need to sleep again. By six months babies might stay awake for two or three hours between sleep periods, and as they reach 12 months will drop some of their daytime sleep as their sleep pressure accumulates more slowly. As all babies are different, there is no ideal window of wakefulness for a particular age, despite what you may see online. Given individual variation and unpredictable changes over time, trying to impose a rigid and unchanging sleep or wake schedule on a baby can be an exercise in futility and frustration. Allowing babies to nap on the go as and when they need to, and trusting the sleep–wake homeostat to ensure they achieve as much sleep as they need to support cognitive development rather than enforcing strict nap times, can be liberating.

Sleep will happen easily for a baby or child when sleep pressure is high, they are in a calm, relaxed state, and nothing is preventing sleep onset. But sometimes babies and children need help to become calm before sleep pressure can kick in and they can nod off.[15] In this situation it can be useful to think about what helps babies become calm and relaxed, and to have a handful of strategies you can use to help your baby unwind. For many babies, physical contact is the preferred option.

One of my PhD students, Lenka Medvecová-Tinková, lives and works in the Czech Republic where she has studied how Czech parents manage bedtime routines for babies and small children. She realized that many parents talked of a concept called ***Uspavani*** that is culturally widespread in Eastern Europe and appears in numerous fairy tales and historical infant care books. Uspavani means to comfort a child to sleep, and while conducting her PhD at Durham University Lenka realized there was no corresponding concept to Uspavani in the English language, nor in the infant sleep literature.[16] So it is unsurprising that parents in English-speaking countries tend to use more distal (noncontact) methods, such as lullabies, music and white noise, to calm babies and help them fall asleep than do Czech parents, who commonly lie with their child, stroke them or cuddle them; physical contact and soothing touch are very effective in dialing down most babies to allow sleep pressure to do its thing. One of the most useful things I figured out when my eldest daughter was a baby was to gently stroke her face from the top of her forehead to the tip of her nose as she was falling asleep. To begin with it was calming and helped her relax so sleep pressure could take over and tip her into sleep—but soon it became a handy sleep association, and for most of her infancy all I had to do when I noticed she was getting sleepy was stroke her face a couple of times and she'd drift right off!

Useful tip

When a baby or young child's sleep pressure is high and the need to sleep is strong, but they are emotionally unable to calm themselves, or they are in a situation where they cannot relax, we may consider them to be "overtired." In this case it is our job as parents to help them become calm, wind down and relax in preparation for sleep. We can do this in many ways. Physical contact such as cuddling, rocking, stroking or patting works for most neurotypical children; actively removing whatever is blocking the action of sleep pressure, such as excitement, fear, pain or anxiety, and helping babies and children to become calm is the simplest way to help them fall asleep.

Babies, then, will sleep whenever their sleep pressure is high enough, so long as any barriers inhibiting sleep are removed. But what happens if we try to make babies fall asleep when their sleep pressure is not high enough? I often hear from parents who are struggling with this issue: they have established a regular bedtime for their babies, which is supported with a routine designed to help the baby relax and learn that sleep time is approaching. But the baby simply will not fall asleep when put into their crib. The same can happen with daytime naps: a pattern has been set up of the baby taking naps at regular times during the day, but at some point, the baby stops falling asleep for a nap as he or she is "supposed to." In both these scenarios parents will sometimes undertake laborious "settling" activities, such as leaning over the crib shushing and patting the baby for long periods of time. Some babies accept the shushing and patting and just lie there, not falling asleep for lengthy periods, as their parents get increasingly fed up. In this situation it is likely that their baby's sleep pressure isn't high enough for them to fall asleep. On other occasions a baby's sleep pressure is high, but shushing and patting are not calming for them, and they mount a strenuous protest. In this case the baby needs help to dial down or unwind, so sleep pressure can be unblocked, which might mean holding or carrying them, feeding them, going for a walk outside, or whatever parents have found works to calm and relax their baby.

In the UK parents often put their babies to bed between 6 and 7 p.m.—we have a bit of a cultural obsession with ensuring small children are in bed and asleep around this time. But for babies, whose sleep patterns change repeatedly throughout the first year as their biological sleep regulators develop and mature, applying this cultural rule rigidly makes little sense. The best "bedtime" for a baby is whenever their sleep pressure is high and their circadian clock is telling them it is sleep time—i.e., when they are biologically ready to fall asleep—and there is no guarantee that this biological tipping point will occur at the same time this week as last week given the rapid brain maturation that occurs over a baby's first year. You might wonder how you are supposed to know when your baby is ready to go to sleep if you don't watch the clock or follow a routine. Simply put, we know they are ready when they start to nod off! Remember, you don't have to be in charge of their sleep—the biological sleep regulators will make sure they get enough sleep, when they need it. Our job is to get out of the way and let them do their work. Trying to *make* babies go to sleep according to a predetermined schedule seems to me to be a pointless exercise in working against their circadian biology and sleep pressure.

> **Useful tip**
>
> If your baby's sleep pressure isn't high, and they are not falling asleep easily despite being relaxed, a change of sleep time and an activity that helps build up sleep pressure may be more effective than persisting with a "settling process" that isn't working.

Understanding that a baby's need for sleep (both in terms of when sleep happens and for how long) can change unpredictably over the first year will save your sanity and protect you from backache caused by leaning over a crib for hours, shushing and patting a baby who is simply not ready to go to sleep. In surviving the first year of parenthood, flexible expectations about baby sleep patterns, trusting their biology, and letting them sleep when they are ready to might be a lot less hassle.

Sleep changes over the first 12 months

As babies mature over time, they can sustain longer wake times between naps as their circadian rhythm matures and they develop a consistent day–night cycle. Consequently, babies start to sleep for longer periods at nighttime, with shorter and fewer sleep bouts during the day. This may begin for some babies around three to four months of age, but for others it may happen later—and all babies will have periods when they resume night-waking, often when they are going through a developmental transition, such as learning to roll or sit, or cutting teeth.

As much as we would like baby sleep development to follow a predictable pattern, this is rarely the case. Sleep development is not a slow, steady progression of babies' longest sleep period gradually increasing night after night—it is more of a roller coaster, with night-waking coming and going over the first few years (which some have labeled "sleep regression," discussed in Chapter 4), and with all babies being on a slightly different track. A similar situation applies when we think about sleep duration, and how much sleep babies need in any 24-hour period.

In a systematic review of 34 published studies of infant sleep duration, Barbara Galland and colleagues in New Zealand found there was hugely variable data for 24-hour sleep averages and their ranges from samples of babies in the first six months of life.[17] In Figure 3.5 we can see the data from Galland's review. The horizontal axis shows the age groups of babies reported in the studies, and the vertical axis shows the number of hours babies slept for. The data points are the average amount of sleep obtained in 24 hours for babies in each study (small black rectangle) and the range (vertical black lines). In the first three months the averages from the 15 studies plotted fall between 12 and 16 hours while the individual babies making up those averages range from 8 to 22 hours. Babies' total sleep time only became consistent across studies and individuals by about one year of age. One thing that parents find very difficult to avoid is comparison: if a friend's baby is sleeping more than your own, could this mean that you are doing something wrong that will somehow compromise your baby's development?

It can be reassuring to know that in the first 12 months very few babies are "average" when it comes to sleep, and while there are all sorts of suggestions and hints made that awful things will befall babies who get insufficient sleep, there is nothing to suggest that healthy babies will sleep too little or too much if we stop interfering and let their biology regulate their sleep duration.

In the months before sleep becomes consolidated at night (which may begin around three to four months of age, but this is variable), sleep–wake patterns can differ considerably between babies. Why some babies appear to sleep through the night and others continue to wake frequently beyond the early months is still poorly understood, and is related to a range of factors that are difficult to assess in infants, such as temperament, irritability and neurodiversity, as well as differences in parental caregiving and possibly even season of birth.[18] Research using overnight video recordings has provided evidence that, although sleep periods lengthen with age, infants continue to wake up during the night throughout the first year of life. In a study using video and parental questionnaire data to examine 100 infants' sleep patterns

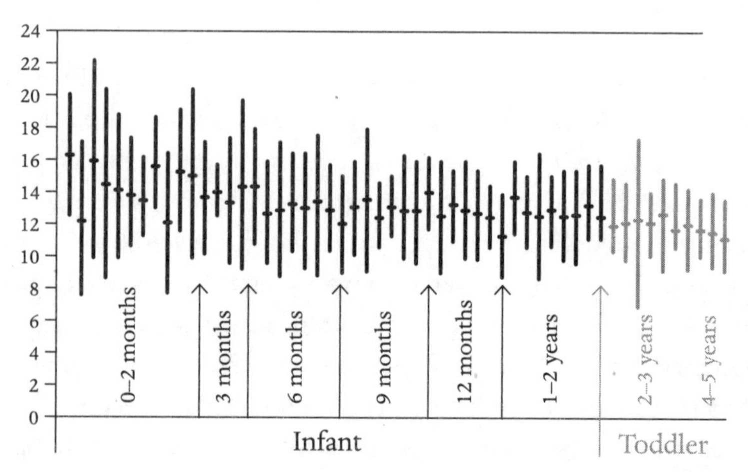

Figure 3.5 24-hour sleep averages and ranges, from Galland et al. (2012)

at five weeks and three months of age, researchers found that a quarter of the babies studied woke and resettled themselves at night, mostly without parental awareness (though this study did not report on how those babies were fed).[19] Another study found that observing babies' behaviors may be only part of the picture.[20] Using EEG monitors on babies, Japanese infant sleep researcher Michiko Yoshida found that some babies who were not showing behavioral signs of being awake were, according to their brain wave activity, awake but not moving. This suggests that what we assume babies are experiencing by observing them from the outside may not be what they are experiencing on the inside, and the assessments of both researchers and parents as to when babies are sleeping and how much sleep they get may be completely inaccurate.

Feeding, contact and comfort

To understand how babies sleep, it can be helpful to think about the biology of other aspects of infant care—such as feeding and contact—and how they might influence the ways in which babies and their parents experience sleep. After all, new parents still receive lots of advice about dropping night feeding and resisting the urge to cuddle their baby "too much." As we have seen, human babies are particularly helpless precocial mammal babies, totally dependent on their caregivers for warmth, safety, comfort and food—none of which they can obtain for themselves during their first year of life, given their lack of strength and poor neuromuscular coordination. Babies' biology is intimately intertwined with, and responsive to, that of their caregivers during this period—and for babies who are breastfed the biological interconnections between a baby and their mother are extensive[21] and can influence sleep behavior in various ways. We will discuss how feed type and sleep patterns are related in detail in Chapter 5, but for now we will focus on how the biology of human milk and lactation affects the biology of human infant sleep.

The milk produced by mothers of precocial mammalian babies generally has a low-fat, high-sugar composition. For most species with precocial babies, the sugar (lactose) supplies the energy needed to cling to or run after their mothers all day long. For baby humans, who have insufficient strength and coordination to cling or run, the high-energy sugar fuels rapid brain growth. Because there is little fat in the milk of precocial species, however, it does not satiate babies for long periods, and so they feed often, day and night.

When they are born, human babies have tiny stomachs, the size of a cherry or a grape. It takes very little milk to fill them up, and they digest it quickly. As your baby grows, their stomach enlarges, but they still cannot consume much milk at each feeding in the first few months. When babies regurgitate milk following a feeding (often known as posseting), this can be a sign that they do not have room in their stomachs for all the milk they have swallowed—this may happen more frequently when babies are given milk from a bottle, as it is more difficult for them to control the flow of milk, how much they consume and when they can stop. When feeding directly at the breast, babies must actively work to extract the milk and take pauses during feeding, so it is easier to stop when they are full.[22] This means that babies fed using bottles can consume more milk than they need—and if this is not human milk, it can take longer for a baby to digest it—leading to the popular practice of giving babies a big bottle of formula before bedtime to "help" them sleep.

It is a common belief that breastfed babies wake more than formula-fed babies, and some parents therefore consider feeding their breastfed baby with formula during the night so that the breastfeeding mother can get more sleep. A growing number of studies have looked for differences in the sleep patterns of breastfed and formula-fed babies and found that there is no difference in the total amount of sleep obtained by feeding type, so long as babies are fed an appropriate amount for their age and size. And while studies confirm that the frequency of awakenings differs—with breastfed babies waking more frequently during the night[23]—research finds that breastfeeding dyads (mother–baby pairs) get the same amount of sleep, or more sleep overall, compared to formula-feeding dyads.[24] This is because, while breastfed babies might wake frequently, neither breastfeeding babies nor their mothers have to wake fully to feed, and they return to sleep more quickly, under the relaxing influence of breastfeeding hormones oxytocin and prolactin, and due to the presence of melatonin—the hormone that promotes sleep—in breast milk. Melatonin is secreted during the night by adults but not by infants. It has a calming effect that promotes sleep, as well as relaxing the smooth muscle of the gastrointestinal tract, allowing for better digestion. Newborn babies who are breastfed during the night therefore benefit from the calming and sleep-inducing effect of melatonin, helping them return to sleep quickly.

But there is another factor at play here. The difference in sleep fragmentation between babies may also be due to differences in mother–baby proximity. Where babies are sleeping—near to their mothers or in a room alone—influences sleeping and feeding patterns. As we know, most newborn babies are intrinsically contact seeking, feeling most relaxed and secure in the arms, or on the body, of a familiar caregiver, and touch is the first of a baby's senses to develop.[25] Skin-to-skin contact after birth is now a staple in many delivery suites (including after C-sections, and with fathers if mothers had general anesthesia), as it is well known that immediate physical contact between mother and baby helps calm babies, helps them thermoregulate, and encourages them to feed early, which simultaneously helps kick-start maternal milk-production.

Although the research on the biological mechanisms for how contact, comfort and touch affect and promote infant sleep is still in its own infancy, the importance of comfort and physical contact for babies' social and emotional development has been recognized for decades. As we saw in Chapter 2, the work of John Bowlby[26] and Harry Harlow[27] on infant attachment emphasized the importance for babies of physical contact and comfort, which has relevance for how babies sleep, but they did not examine the biology of touch and how it calms babies. A growing body of evidence on the importance of touch is beginning to explain why babies find contact and touch pleasurable, calming, relaxing and sleep promoting. The bottom line is that physical contact and touch are extremely important in helping babies to relax, and very useful tools for helping them dial down sufficiently to fall asleep.

What is important to know is that needing to feed frequently night and day is normal for human babies, not just in the first days and weeks but for several months. Parents develop different ways of dealing with the interruption to their own sleep, which we will explore in later chapters, as this is consistently the aspect of early parenthood that new parents find most difficult. I often hear from parents who are desperate to know when sleep will "improve," or whose search for a quick fix has left them even more frustrated. I reassure them that if they can go with the flow, anticipate that nighttime will be fragmented for at least a few months and possibly much longer, and—where possible—ask for and accept help from family and friends when they need it, they will manage. Some nights will be difficult and some less so. When they are anticipating their baby will sleep, wake, seek contact, and feed frequently night and day for the first few months, they find this period in their baby's life much less difficult.

Useful tips

- In the early days remember that your baby will sleep in many short bouts with no day–night rhythm. Feeding and contact will help them fall asleep. Wait until they are floppy before you try to put them down.
- As they reach the end of the Fourth Trimester (three months), watch for the buildup of sleep pressure and help them relax so sleep pressure can do its thing. No one can fall asleep on command, and babies are no exception.
- Help your baby's circadian clock develop by taking them outside in the morning and keeping them in the daylight with the noise of normal activities during the day. While you can't force your baby's sleep to fit around your schedule, you can let them sleep on the go, as and when they need to, so you aren't tied to the house and their sleep–wake schedule.

Key things to remember about baby sleep biology

Sleep biology may seem complex because it involves multiple biological systems, but when you grasp how these work, sleep is straightforward and predictable. With babies, an added complication is that the systems mature at different rates in different babies, because biological variation exists. So it is important to have realistic and flexible expectations for how baby-sleep biology unfolds, and how variable it can be. It is helpful to be aware of general developmental trends over time, but resist the urge to benchmark them against specific weeks or months—every baby develops at their own rate, and this variation is completely normal. As we will discover in the next chapter, when it comes to baby-sleep development, biological variability is the norm, and both cultural and statistical normalcy can be misleading.

4. Normal is as normal does

Although I am an academic researcher and neither a medical doctor nor a wizard, people sometimes think I might have a magic wand or potion with which I can "fix" their babies' sleep. Many questions I receive begin along the lines of "I don't think my baby's sleep is normal. . . ." Other parents might suspect their baby's sleep is pretty typical, but they have been rattled by someone's comment or something they've read and want me to eliminate their concerns. Most of the questions I am asked are variations on a handful of themes, which begin with: I am worried that...

> ...my baby isn't sleeping how I, my partner, my mom, my friend, someone on Instagram thinks they should. What should I do?
>
> ...my baby isn't doing what my sister's, friend's, cousin's, random acquaintance's baby is doing. How do I make my baby do this?
>
> ...someone online said that what I am doing (using a sling, a pacifier, swaddling, rocking, etc.) is not good for my baby. Are they right?
>
> ...a blog I read said what I am doing (responding in the night, bed-sharing, keeping baby downstairs until we go to bed) will cause problems. Is that true?
>
> ...I don't actually know what I am doing and there is so much conflicting information. I need help.

In these situations, parents usually want reassurance that nothing is wrong with their baby, that their baby's behavior is normal, or that what they are doing is not harmful. I always point out that if they are concerned their baby is unwell, they should consult a relevant health professional, but I also reassure them that when it comes to infant sleep behavior over the first year, there is a very wide range of normal.

It can be helpful to think about how our evolutionary legacies, and our basic sleep biology, can inform realistic expectations for how babies sleep and offer reassurance when you are worried about what is and isn't "normal," and whether you are "doing the wrong thing." Ways of "managing" infant sleep are different all around the world, and exposure to different ways of doing things can offer new insights. This information can also help us understand how the science of baby sleep in Western settings has been shaped by the historical, political and cultural contexts in which it has been carried out, and how many of the misalignments between the biology of baby humans and culturally developed expectations that feed parental anxieties have arisen.

When we are trying to understand how babies sleep, understanding parents' anxieties is, in my view, crucial. Parental anxieties are not only very common, but they can also be contagious, and are often detected and amplified by babies who cannot relax and be comforted when their parents are stressed or tense, creating a vicious cycle that perpetuates babies' unsettled behavior and fuels further parental concern. Oftentimes breaking this cycle with reassurance that a baby's desire for contact, need for frequent feedings, or tendency to wake during the night is typical and expected behavior for most baby humans is all that is needed.

What is "normal" infant sleep?

I have spent the past 30 years contemplating how people understand the concept of "normal" infant sleep. Although many people claim to know what this might look like, their explanations are wildly different, and as we have seen they can be heavily influenced by historical and cultural expectations, and reinforced by how their own infants conformed to or contradicted these embedded beliefs.

When parents ask "is my baby's sleep normal?," they usually want to know "is my baby doing what s/he should be doing" or "is my baby the same as other babies?" The first interpretation presumes there is some kind of "gold standard" against which babies' sleep should be measured, and parents are seeking a benchmark with which they can assess their baby's sleep behavior. The second interpretation assumes babies are homogenous and all behave in the same way, and parents want to know whether their baby is an outlier. But both interpretations are problematic as there is no "universal standard" for baby sleep, nor is there a "standard baby" that can be used as a universal comparator. Because there are historical and social expectations embedded in every culture that are passed on in myths, sayings and culture-specific rules, new parents in many Western societies often feel their baby must measure up to (what in my opinion is) an unhealthy cultural obsession with "normal infant sleep." This perceived pressure provokes parents' anxiety and causes them to think that they could or should be doing something differently—or that there is something they are not doing (or buying)—that would help their baby fall asleep more quickly, sleep longer, or more deeply, or through the night.[1] Sleep product manufacturers, advertisers, television producers, influencers and social media commentators have a lot to answer for!

Studies confirm the role that culture plays in shaping these anxieties. In western English-speaking countries (UK, U.S., Australia, etc.), the proportion of parents who report that their baby has a "**sleep problem**" is high: 25–30 percent is the commonly reported statistic.[2] However, when similar studies are conducted in non-Western industrialized countries such as Japan and Korea, the proportion of parents reporting their baby has a "sleep problem" is typically around 5–7 percent.[3] Korean and Japanese babies are not biologically better sleepers than babies born in the U.S. or UK; biologically, all human babies are born with undeveloped brains and go through the same processes of maturation and development. The reason such differences are seen in parents' reports of infant sleep problems is that those things UK and U.S. parents find problematic about their babies' sleep—frequent night-waking and contact seeking—are accepted aspects of baby behavior in countries such as Korea and Japan. As a result, parents perceive their babies differently.[4]

During her postdoctoral fellowship at Durham University, my colleague Dr. Alanna Rudzik (now associate professor of anthropology at SUNY Oneonta) ran a series of focus groups with mothers about their experiences with babies' sleep. Mothers who took part in the focus groups were of different ages, ethnicities and socioeconomic backgrounds, yet most felt "under pressure" to ensure their babies' sleep behaviors met social expectations. This pressure came from partners, family members, friends, parenting guidebooks, the internet and social media, traditional media and health professionals. (In later chapters we will think about how this perceived pressure to make a baby conform to cultural and historical norms affects parental well-being, but for now we will focus on its consequences for babies.)

When their babies' sleep behaviors do not meet their own or other people's expectations, parents may begin to question whether their baby has a sleep problem that they must somehow fix.[5] What Alanna and I wanted to understand was how UK parents identify that their baby has a sleep problem. We wanted to explore the ways in which the conflict between social expectations and babies' biologically driven needs and behaviors are experienced and managed within families.[6]

We found that three ways of understanding "normality" were commonly used in discussions of babies' sleep: what's biologically expectable, what's socially desirable, and what's statistically prevalent. Some mothers emphasized biological normalcy by describing their babies' needs and what's "natural" for babies. One participant emphasized that babies sleep when they need to, and parents have to work around them. Other mothers reflected social or cultural normalcy in describing how babies "should" behave, such as sleeping when they are expected to and being "in a routine." In other cases, mothers invoked statistical normalcy when they referenced average "milestones" for baby sleep, articulating benchmarks such as "At three months they should have started sleeping through," and "I'm dreading next month 'cos she'll be dropping a nap, and it'll all go haywire."

As we have seen, the biological norm relates to the fundamental mammalian physiology of the mother–baby dyad: the mother's body stabilizing the baby's temperature, the baby's feeding attempts triggering the mother to lactate, the hormones in the mother's milk and the act of suckling causing the baby to feel sleepy, the soporific effect of feeding hormones on the mother, the need of human babies to feed frequently to fuel their growing brain, the need of mothers to feed their babies frequently to sustain milk production, the synchronization of mother–baby sleep cycles and their mutual responsiveness during shared sleep. Alanna and I found aspects of this being mentioned by some mothers in our focus groups around a decade ago, who simply brought their babies into bed when they wanted to nurse frequently and found this allowed them to feed and sleep with minimal disruption. While this perspective was not commonly discussed in the UK in the mid- to late nineties, when my colleagues and I were initially interviewing parents about their experiences of baby sleep, it is now often used by midwives, doulas, infant feeding professionals, and by some infant sleep educators, indicating that the evidence around how maternal–infant physiology and behavior work took 20 years to filter through to parents (more on this in Chapters 5 and 6).

In contrast, it is primarily historical and cultural views of what is "normal" (with a sprinkling of politics and religion) that shape public discourse and perceptions of infant sleep within our society. These ideas reflect the underlying beliefs about baby sleep that are embedded in specific cultural groups. They are a product of specific historical influences, sociopolitical changes, and responses to past ecological or economic needs, and have been heavily influenced by the views and practices of wealthy Western "elites," self-appointed experts, product advertising and media sensationalism.

We reinforce these views between ourselves when we ask friends and family if their newborn is a "good baby," or whether their young baby is "sleeping through the night." Changing the cultural narrative to inquire of new parents how they are coping with their baby's frequent night-waking, and whether we can do anything to help them in any way, would go a long way to normalizing the practical challenges of early parenthood and the need for support.

Epidemiological, public health and clinical recommendations are founded on concepts of statistical normalcy, such as the average or the normative range produced across various studies.

Statistical norms using measures of central tendency—such as means or medians—are assumed to reflect the sleep behaviors of the majority of babies, but as the last chapter illustrated, there is a huge range of variation within and between the studies used to generate measures of statistical normalcy, and there is a great deal of bias in terms of which babies have been studied, and therefore which populations those averages are based on. It is worth exploring this in more detail.

Defining "normal"

I was ten when my brother was born (in the early seventies), so my younger sister and I would sometimes accompany him and our mom on their trips to the weekly baby clinic to be weighed. This to me was an odd experience: the baby clinic was held in our Methodist chapel hall, which was where we went every week for Sunday school. To transform the space from Sunday school to baby clinic, the staff would section off areas with green fabric screens on wheels and set out noticeboards containing information for parents to read. This included charts and tables of typical baby weights and normal developmental stages.[7] I would look at these charts at every visit to see what to expect from my baby brother next: Should he be sitting soon, or crawling or standing? In those days, measuring up to the charts was a competitive business. "How's yours doing?" one mom would ask another while they were sitting on the row of chairs in the "waiting area" for their turn to see the health visitor (who they called the "nurse"). I heard mothers whose babies weren't "keeping up" receive sympathetic murmurs from others, but also heard their judgment when those mothers whose babies were not measuring up to the "norms" left the clinic.

Two decades later, when I had my own children, the church hall baby clinics had long gone, and there were no charts on the wall of the local GP surgery where we took our babies for their immunizations. The statistical norms were less prominently displayed but could still be found as charts and tables in parent-facing leaflets and self-help parenting books detailing "What to Expect" and "Your baby's first year." Today, health professionals (at least in the UK) track most developmental milestones according to a baby's own individual trajectory in their "Red Book"[8] rather than in comparison to a standard norm found in a chart or table—however, such graphs and charts are still found on websites and are particularly prominent in phone apps that are marketed for parents to track their babies' biological functions and development.[9] Whatever form they take, these charts, tables and milestone reminders often include recommendations or guidelines for baby sleep duration at different ages (see Figure 4.1).

Let's stop and think about these "sleep schedules" for a moment. What does a chart, table or phone app displaying the "recommended sleep duration" for your baby really mean? What are those recommended hours of sleep based on?

Many parents assume that these "recommendations" or "guidelines" for baby sleep duration are based on research studies that have assessed how much sleep a "typical" baby needs for "optimal development" (if such a thing exists)—but this is not the case. They are based on the normative values for baby sleep at different ages generated by one or more studies. Charts, tables and apps of recommended sleep duration therefore only tell you how long other babies were reported to sleep at another place and time. And many of the reference studies used to generate these normative values: a) were conducted 50 to 70 years ago; and b) recruited mostly Western white middle-class and well-educated parents, whose babies were raised in particular cultural contexts in which

Source	Age	Day Sleep	Night Sleep	Total Sleep
Baby Centre[10]	0 months	8–9 hours	8 hours	16 hours
	1 month	8 hours	9 hours	17 hours
	3 months	6 hours	10 hours	16 hours
	6 months	5 hours	10 hours	15 hours
	9 months	3.5 hours	11 hours	14.5 hours
	12 months	3 hours	11 hours	14 hours
Happiest Baby[11]	0–2 months	6–8 hours	8–10 hours	14–18 hours
	2–4 months	4–6 hours	8–10 hours	12–16 hours
	4–12 months	3–5 hours	9–11 hours	12–16 hours
Bibino app[12]	0–1 month	3–4.5 hours	2–4 hours	14–18 hours
	1–2 months	2.25–5 hours	4–6 hours	11–15 hours
	2–4 months	2.25–8 hours	6–8 hours	12–14 hours
	4–8 months	2–6 hours	6–12 hours	12–14 hours
	8–12 months	2–4 hours	10–12 hours	12–14 hours

Figure 4.1 Recommended sleep "schedules" for ages 0–12 months from popular online sources

infant care options (e.g., feeding methods, sleep locations, etc.) reflected specific cultural beliefs.[13] Recommended sleep durations for babies, then, tell you nothing about the sleep needs of *your* baby for "optimal development"—they tell you only the average amount of sleep obtained by other babies (whose developmental outcomes are unknown) in studies that may or may not have any contextual relevance to you or your child.

Studying sleep "norms"

How, then, have researchers examined infant sleep, and what do their studies tell us? The earliest scientific studies of infant sleep published in the mid-twentieth century followed the prevailing model of adult sleep research in studying "convenience samples" of volunteers (usually students).[14] In the emerging field of infant sleep research, participants were recruited from families to whom clinicians and researchers had easy access (often their own, their friends' and colleagues'). Statistical "norms" for baby sleep were therefore defined based on studies of relatively well-off, Western white babies. Following the middle-class trends of the period, these babies were predominantly fed infant formula, slept in a room on their own at night, and were placed **prone** (chest down) for sleep.[15] The conditions in which these babies lived and slept differed substantially from those of today's babies, and indeed from babies throughout the evolutionary history of the human species. This means that despite being widely quoted, these studies have limited relevance today.

A prominent example that claimed to "define normal infant sleep," and that has been heavily cited in baby books, pediatric textbooks and clinical recommendations, was conducted in the 1950s by pioneer infant sleep researchers Moore and Ucko. They remarked that 50 percent of the six-month-old English babies they studied exhibited "problematic night-waking."[16] This was the beginning of the concept that babies can have "sleep problems" that are defined by causing sleep disruption for their parents. The notion that night-waking constitutes "an infant sleep problem," parentally defined, is now widespread in many Western settings.

Moore and Ucko's study aimed to document "normal sleep development" by studying 160 babies who belonged to a group of 200 "central London families" taking part in a longitudinal cohort study. In so doing they created a definition of "sleeping through the night" that has been misunderstood and misused by parents and practitioners ever since. In Moore and Ucko's study, for no clearly explicable reason, a baby was deemed to "sleep through the night" when the parents reported the baby did not cry or fuss between midnight and 5 a.m. In addition to "sleeping through the night," data collected via maternal report were analyzed to determine the age at which each baby first "settled" (began regularly "sleeping through the night," as per their definition) and their general tendency to wake at night during any given period.

Of the 160 babies Moore and Ucko studied, 70 percent stopped waking in the night (were not reported to cry or fuss between midnight and 5 a.m.) around the age of three months—and soon it became the advice of clinicians and the goal of parents that infants *should settle* (begin sleeping through the night) by three months of age.[17] At the time, tables cataloging babies' month-by-month sleep development were hugely popular. However, Moore and Ucko's paper also reported that although 70 percent of babies "settled" around three months of age, at least half of "early settlers" resumed night-waking during their fourth month, but this piece of contextual information—which is hugely important for helping parents create realistic expectations—was not reported in textbooks and baby-care manuals at the time. The selectively chosen results of Moore and Ucko's study quickly became regarded as normative milestones against which all babies' sleep could or should be measured. Following the rediscovery of Moore and Ucko's study a decade or so ago, the phenomenon of babies resuming night-waking at four months after a spell of sleep consolidation has become known (unhelpfully) in the parenting literature as the "four-month sleep regression" (see discussion later in this chapter).

Nearly fifty years after Moore and Ucko, Dr. Jacki Henderson, now a senior lecturer in developmental psychology at the University of Canterbury in Christchurch, New Zealand, revisited their definition of "sleeping through the night" for her PhD research. She investigated infant sleep consolidation over the first year of life in 75 middle-income, predominantly white New Zealand families whose babies were healthy, born at term and developing typically.[18] She used three criteria for "sleeping through the night": the first was Moore and Ucko's five-hour period of 12–5 a.m.; the second was "any unbroken eight-hour stretch" (as parents tended to want their babies to sleep for eight rather than five hours); and the third was a "family congruent" definition that reflected the actual eight-hour period parents considered as "sleeping through the night": 10 p.m. to 6 a.m.[19] Data were reported by parents who completed sleep diaries for six days each month for 12 months, reporting (among other things) all "sustained awakenings" of more than two minutes. Henderson assessed the accuracy of parents' sleep diary reports using video for 40 percent of the sleeping babies and found a high level of agreement across the measures (93–97%).

She examined the data to: a) assess at what age babies met each of the criteria for sleeping through the night; b) compare babies' abilities to meet these criteria; and c) identify when the majority did so. To be judged as consistently "sleeping through the night," a baby had to meet the specified criteria for five out of the six nights reported.

The biggest increase in sleep consolidation happened between one and four months of age. More than 50 percent of babies met criterion 1—sleeping from 12–5 a.m.—between three and four months (58%); criterion 2—sleeping for an unbroken eight-hour stretch—between four and five months (58%); and criterion 3—sleeping from 10 p.m. to 6 a.m.—between five and six months (53%). Between six and nine months there was a small increase in the proportion of babies who met each of the criteria, and by the time they were 12 months of age 87 percent, 86 percent, and 73 percent of babies were "sleeping through the night" according to criteria 1, 2 and 3, respectively, meaning 13 percent, 14 percent and 27 percent were not doing so.[20]

While this study provides some useful insights into baby sleep development, there are some factors that limit the generalizability of the results. First, the participants did not fully represent the local population in terms of ethnicity and socioeconomic diversity, meaning that data from families with different beliefs and practices regarding baby sleep, such as **bed-sharing** among Maori and Pacific Islander families, were not included. Second, study dropouts may have been more likely to have babies with regulatory problems, and so the outcomes reported may reflect a biased sample—that is to say, this sample might represent babies more likely to "sleep through," according to all three definitions, and not be a truly representative sample. The key take-home message from this study for me was that individual babies are on very different trajectories: in this sample of 75 mainly white middle-income New Zealand babies, around half slept from 10 p.m. to 6 a.m. without disrupting their parents while the other half didn't. And while two-thirds slept "through the night" after 12 months of age, almost one-third had never yet done so.

Henderson's study reinforces the picture that baby sleep development is variable and individual throughout the first year of life, and for the most part it is impossible for parents to predict how their baby's sleep development will unfold. Sleep patterns are certainly very different from one baby to the next within the same family—many parents recount stories of how they genuinely felt they had "cracked it" with their first child, who caused minimal nighttime disruption, only to be blindsided by their second child, who woke frequently throughout the entire first year. For other families the story is reversed. In most of these cases the sleep and care environments are consistent, but the babies have different temperaments, regulatory abilities or sleep needs.

Useful tip

Don't pin your hopes on your baby sleeping through the night at two or three or four months, or at any given age. If they do, view it as a bonus!

Normalized expectations

An issue that has been investigated in multiple studies of infant sleep development as a potential cause of sleep disruption is infant feed type. We do not know from Henderson's study whether the babies who showed early sleep consolidation were more likely to be fed formula versus breast milk, or whether their parents introduced solid foods from an early age.[21] We will explore the research findings on feeding and sleeping in detail in the next chapter; however, it is worth noting here that although Moore and Ucko recognized that feeding breast milk or formula could have an impact upon infant sleep behavior, the establishment of prolonged and early sleep habits were their principal priority, noting that "weaning to a bottle or complementary feeds sometimes had an immediate beneficial effect on sleep."

It is not difficult to see, given such statements, where many popularly expressed notions about baby sleep come from, and as decades passed (and to the detriment of breastfeeding) the pursuit of early and unbroken sleep in young infants became a parental priority. Expectations regarding the "normal" pattern of infant sleep development in the English-speaking world were embedded in pediatric and parenting manuals, culminating in authoritative statements at the end of the twentieth century, such as the second sentence in the opening paragraph of the American Academy of Pediatrics' *Guide to Your Child's Sleep*, which states: "In early infancy, the first task is to help your baby learn to sleep longer at night. . . ."[22] As an anthropologist my first reaction is "why?" Why must babies learn to sleep through the night in early infancy? Why is helping their baby accomplish this considered a parent's first task? And why is such a statement made by a highly credentialed clinical organization?

We've already discussed some of the answers to these questions: a) because the historical and cultural background of the United States (and other countries) has created a situation where adult needs are emphasized and babies are expected to comply with them from as early an age as possible; b) because the baby's biological needs for comfort, warmth, food and safety receive minimal or no recognition in contexts where parents are expected to prioritize their roles in economic production over their roles in reproduction; and c) because the clinical specialty of pediatrics in the U.S. has been shaped by the ideals of capitalism, independence and self-sufficiency, which color the lenses through which the role of parents is viewed by many clinicians. Unfortunately, given the prestige and reach of such institutions, their contextually specific statements are often taken up and implemented far beyond their jurisdiction, into settings where traditional cultural practices and beliefs are doing babies no harm and causing parents no anxiety, but are swept aside because they are considered "old-fashioned."

Cross-cultural perspectives on "normal" infant sleep

Although all babies' sleep biology works in the same way, people from different countries or cultural backgrounds have very different expectations of baby sleep, and very different practices around nighttime infant care.

For instance, first-generation Pakistani mothers in Bradford (a multiethnic city in the north of England) are clear that they would never leave their babies alone to sleep during the daytime. This, they told us in a 2016 study, is something they know that "the English mothers" do, but "a Pakistani mother would never leave her baby alone by themselves upstairs." One emphasized, "she is always with me. I like to have her with me." "We rarely put him down," said another, "someone is always holding him, there are always several of us here, so someone can always hold him." At nighttime they described communal sleeping, with parents and children all in the same room. Babies shared a bed with their mothers while fathers often had a separate bed, or shared with older children. "He don't mind," said one interviewee about her husband, "it's only babies, and a good Pakistani father expects that."[23]

In contrast, English women in the same Bradford neighborhoods described how they frequently put their babies upstairs on their own in a crib during the daytime (contrary to infant sleep safety guidelines, see Chapter 7). One described this as being for her daughter's benefit, "so she can get a bit of nice sleep, where it's quiet." Another added that "It's good for me to have him up there—gives me time to get stuff done, like housework and that." At night, many of the English babies slept in their parents' rooms for a couple of months, but by three months were being moved into their own room to sleep. "My husband said it were time he went in his own room," said one. Another put their baby in a room alone from the first night home from the hospital: "We done it all out and it's lovely in there for him," this interviewee reported, "and this way we don't disturb him, and he don't disturb us."[24] For both cultural groups, their behaviors around daytime and nighttime baby sleep were quite normal—they were doing what they believed most people like them were also doing: normal is as normal does.

These interviews with Pakistani and English mothers were conducted by another of my PhD students, Dr. Denise Crane, as part of the Born in Bradford (BiB) Project.[25] Denise interviewed 46 new mothers, all enrolled in BiB, who invited her into their homes and shared insights into their lives. She found that living in multigenerational households in the UK enabled first-generation Pakistani women to care for their babies much as they would have in their birth country, with an extended network of family or in-laws on hand to provide support. However, second- and third-generation Pakistani women she spoke to (those who were born in the UK, or whose parents were born here, and who identified themselves as British Pakistani) described lives much like the other English-born participants.

The strategies new mothers employed to cope with baby care and to manage daily life reflected the cultural pressures, personal expectations, and opportunities for support they experienced. Maternal isolation (particularly from extended family) was associated with encouraging babies to sleep alone and attempting to foster sleep independence from an early age, much as John B. Watson– and Frederick Truby King–era mothers had done, in an effort to give themselves time to devote to other tasks. The support of relatives who were close at hand was associated with communal and responsive infant care.

Useful tip

Asking friends and relatives for practical support during the first year of your baby's life can be a game-changer. What you ask them to do need not be complicated. In the newborn phase it can be sufficient to simply make you a cup of coffee (and fill a flask with more for later) and provide something nutritious to eat while you are in the frequent-feeding phase. Or, if you need to nap, they could take your baby out for a walk. With an older baby they could simply come and hold him or her while you take a break or catch up on chores. Don't underestimate the value of the mental break you'll get from having another pair of eyes and hands on an inquisitive 10-month old!

While anthropologists have been aware of cultural differences in infant care practices, in the world of infant sleep research the variability of baby sleep practices was rarely acknowledged until the internet made it easy to collect online survey data from around the world. Online survey studies have lots of limitations, of course, as it is impossible to control who they reach or who completes them once they are unleashed into the online universe, so we should be cautious of drawing definitive conclusions from them.[26] But they can be useful for illustrating differences in beliefs and practices, and have highlighted some dramatic cross-country differences that are worth mentioning (with a proverbial grain of salt).

In one large and often-cited online survey, almost 30,000 people (presumed to be parents) completed a baby/toddler sleep survey.[27] The respondents lived in 17 large urban communities around the world (Australia, Canada, China, Hong Kong, India, Indonesia, Korea, Japan, Malaysia, New Zealand, Philippines, Singapore, Taiwan, Thailand, United Kingdom, United States, and Vietnam), grouped for comparative purposes into "Asian" and "Western."[28] In Asian countries babies and toddlers had later bedtimes, later rise times, less nighttime sleep and less total sleep than in "Western" countries. Bedtimes for babies and toddlers across the 17 locations varied by almost three hours, from half-past seven in New Zealand to quarter-past ten in Hong Kong, and nighttime sleep duration varied by 1 hour and 40 minutes (11.6 hours in Japan to 13.3 hours in New Zealand), but there were minimal differences in daytime sleep.

Parents' perceptions of whether their babies experienced "sleep problems" also varied widely, as did the degree of parental involvement in helping babies and young children fall asleep and stay asleep.[29] Very few (4%) children living in "Asian" countries, but many more (57%) in "Western" countries, were expected to fall asleep independently (that is, without a parent or caregiver present). Likewise, very few (2%) parents in "Asian" countries allowed their child to cry themselves to sleep, in comparison with over 15 percent of "Western" parents. This is strongly related to the fact that in "Asian" countries babies and children are much more likely to bed-share (65%) or room-share (88%) with their parents than in "Western" countries (where 12% bed-sharing and 22% room-sharing was reported). Although the authors state that they designed the study with the intention of capturing data about equal numbers of babies in various age brackets from each country surveyed, they do not report whether they actually accomplished this, and so the results may reflect skewed age distributions.

While online surveys can offer us a broad sense of how sleep patterns and nighttime parenting differ from place to place, they offer very little insight into why people in different places have different sleeping and parenting habits, and what these differences might mean. So let's close this chapter by exploring some of the ethnographic studies of baby sleep in different cultures to understand how the various approaches are explained, and why cultural differences are important.

Ethnographic insights on how babies sleep

Although the early ethnographers mostly ignored the lives of mothers and babies, over the past twenty years a few have taken up the challenge of conducting ethnographies of baby care. Dr. Alma Gottlieb's study of childcare practices among the Beng people of Côte d'Ivoire in West Africa included a detailed account of mother–baby sleep.[30] She found little regimentation of when babies slept or fed among the Beng, and no bedtimes or bedtime routines. Beng mothers were not anxious about their babies' sleep, it just happened. Mothers and others carried babies during regular daily activities with babies falling asleep and waking as the need arose. At night the cloth with which babies were held during the day was untied, and babies breastfed and fell asleep next to their mothers. Nighttime mother–baby **co-sleeping** was the cultural norm, and breastfeeding and infant sleep were intimately intertwined.

Meanwhile, in her study of Japanese families, Diana Tahhan describes how co-sleeping is believed necessary by both men and women to ensure physical safety in case of emergencies and to facilitate not just caregiving, but overall well-being.[31] In exploring the sense of safety, security and reassurance—*anshinkan*—that shared sleep produces for parents as well as their children, Tahhan found that Japanese sleep practices reproduce and embody cultural values of closeness between parents and children. She highlights the importance of intimacy through touch within families, or "skinship," as well as the inter-embodied experience that results from parent–infant co-sleeping, which establishes and maintains interconnection even once the child moves out of the parental room.

These detailed ethnographic studies reinforce accounts of

infant care in widespread locations such as Guatemala, Italy, Spain and rural U.S. Among Mayan families in Guatemala, babies commonly fall asleep in someone's arms and are taken to bed with their parents, sleeping with their mothers from birth to two or three years of age, or until the birth of their next sibling. Here, sleeping alone is undesirable, and mothers responded with shock and disapproval at the American custom of leaving babies in rooms on their own. Mayan mothers "cannot conceive of any other way to sleep their baby than by their side—and in fact some argue that to separate an infant from its mother for sleep is abusive or neglectful treatment."[32]

This is not an uncommon point of view. As previously noted, Italian parents were critical of the American norm of putting children to bed in separate rooms.[33] Similar observations were made by ethnographers in the Basque region of Spain.[34] Even within America, some cultural subgroups embrace traditional infant sleep practices that run counter to the dominant child-rearing ideology. Susan Abbott's ethnography of rural Appalachian families in Eastern Kentucky, for instance, emphasized how—as in Japan—family solidarity was reinforced by physical sleep contact during infancy and childhood.[35] A similar sense of closeness and reassurance is described by Cook Islanders in the Pacific.[36]

In contrast, my colleague Dr. Cecilia Tomori's ethnography of nighttime caregiving and breastfeeding in an American midwestern town highlights how expectant parents spend considerable time and effort during pregnancy preparing a nursery—a separate room, centered around a crib, where their baby is expected to sleep independently without contact with their parents.[37] Soon after birth, however, she describes how the participants in her study had to confront the reality that breastfed babies fall asleep while feeding, and when put down in the crib, do not stay asleep. Prior to the birth of their baby, U.S. parents seemed to be unaware of the fact that babies often need physical contact for comfort and to relax enough to be able to fall asleep. Cecilia documented how parents negotiated the various dilemmas caused by the conflict between babies' needs and parents' expectations around feeding and sleeping, which often fueled parents' stress, which their baby then responded to. The dilemmas and tensions experienced by parents around sleep and sleep recommendations in Western settings can cause parents to pursue medical treatment for babies who are simply seeking the contact and calm reassurance that Beng, Mayan, Japanese, South Pacific, rural Appalachian and the Pakistani babies in Bradford experience as part of the culture of everyday baby care.

Dr. Vicky Thomas is a consultant pediatrician and friend of mine who runs a weekly clinic in the UK for "unsettled babies" referred by GPs or health visitors following parents' concerns that "something" is wrong with their baby—difficulty settling to sleep, staying asleep, prolonged crying, or "refusal" to be put down. When parents share their concerns in her clinic, she asks what they are hoping the outcome of the consultation will be. Generally, parents are looking for "a treatment" (such as medication or prescription formula) to help their baby's digestion/colic/reflux/other problems and improve sleep—basically to "settle" their baby and reduce the disruption to their own sleep. The treatments that are prescribed typically take a couple of weeks to show an effect, and Vicky warns parents that they should not expect overnight results. As her clinic is held on Thursdays, five days later she will call the families she has seen to follow-up. Regularly, parents report that everything is much improved, the treatment has worked, the baby is more settled, and the parents are feeling relieved (and sleeping better). Yet the prescription just does not work this fast. The most effective thing Vicky does, she says, is listen to their concerns, validate them, and provide reassurance, ensuring they feel heard by a medical professional who understands they are distressed and has taken action to improve the situation. Having been heard, the parents generally begin to relax and feel less anxious—and consequently so does their baby.

Unsettled, irritable, frequently waking babies who are constantly seeking parental contact or who have difficulty relaxing enough to fall or stay asleep may be responding to the stress and anxiety radiating from their parents, and reassurance can help reset the relationship. Of course, some babies do have an underlying medical condition, but these are much less frequent than is often believed.[38] The best thing you can do to improve your baby's sleep—and your own—might simply be to stop trying to improve it.

Useful tip

Accept your baby's need for contact and comfort: hold them, cuddle them, carry them in a sling or soft carrier if that is helpful.[39] Babies are adept at responding if you are stressed by dialing themselves up, thus making the stress worse. Try to find ways to calm yourself and you'll likely find your baby will become calmer too.

How popular trends influence our perception of "normal"

I have been observing babies, their parents and sleep science now for several decades, and have had the opportunity to notice new tumbleweeds roll across the baby sleep landscape. A particularly prominent one of these is the notion of "sleep regression," which was first mentioned in parenting guides 20 or so years ago, and which now appears to have become normalized within parent-talk. Almost all new parents have now heard of (and most are dreading) the "four-month sleep regression," while many claim there are multiple other sleep regressions to be aware of too. When I was a new mother, sleep regressions were not a thing—so I wondered where they came from, and what evidence gave rise to their normalcy in the expectations of today's parents. But, despite searching multiple databases of scientific and clinical research articles, I could find no studies relating to sleep regression. The term simply doesn't exist within the scientific evidence base on baby sleep, even though internet search engines such as Google, Bing and Yahoo return dozens of hits in blogs, websites and media articles.

It seems that the notion of "sleep regression" was invented and normalized within self-help infant-care literature, with sleep coaches and authors of advice for parents amplifying the notion that at four months (and possibly eight months and 18 months), sleep disruption is a given. These "regressions" are often linked to significant growth spurts, developmental changes, or new skills that a baby is learning (sometimes labeled "leaps"), which can temporarily disrupt their sleep routines; "regressions" do not happen to all babies, they do not occur with predictable timing, they are not a recognized component of baby sleep biology, and they do not mean that a baby's sleep is "regressing" or going backward. As I have previously mentioned, baby sleep development is not a linear process where unbroken nighttime sleep gets progressively longer and longer; it is much more like a roller coaster where sleep disruption comes and goes periodically throughout the first year and beyond, happening at different times for different babies.

While the notion of sleep regression *may* have begun as a

"heads-up" to parents to avoid becoming complacent about their three-month-old's newfound ability to consolidate sleep into longer stretches at night, and to offer a warning that many babies resume night-waking, it has taken on the mantle of a predictable component of baby sleep biology, which it is not, but neither is it a "sleep problem." Rather than fearing the next "regression," try to accept the sleep disruption roller coaster as an inevitable part of the first year with a new baby, and reach out for support from alloparents during the rough spots.

Key things to remember about "normality"

If you are worried that your baby's sleep may not be "normal" and feel that you need to do something to help your baby sleep longer, deeper or through the night, be reassured that this is a very common feeling among new parents. But be aware that comparing your baby's sleep development to that of others—or to data that claims to represent the "average" baby—can cause anxiety or stress that your baby might respond to by becoming tense or irritable. Knowing the different ways in which "normal" can be understood can help parents accept that their baby is developing according to his or her own trajectory. It is also helpful to keep in mind that your baby's sleep behavior at any one time doesn't necessarily predict what their sleep might be like next week, next month or next year. Parents' strategies and ideas will often change across the first year of their baby's life, and it is important to be open to experimenting to find out what works for you and your baby (which may well be different from what worked for your friend or sister, or from your older children). And remember that what we think of as "normal" depends on who we are, what ideas we have been exposed to, our vantage point—and this applies to parents, clinicians and sleep experts alike.

As we have seen, popular beliefs about baby sleep can be laden with historical and cultural baggage, exacerbated by a limited understanding of sleep biology. When well-meaning friends and relatives suggest that you should "teach" your baby to sleep through the night from an early age, such advice is unhelpful and unnecessary. Asking new parents if they have a "good baby" implies there is something wrong if their baby is not sleeping 24/7, and though friends and family might not be aware of it, asking such questions can cause anxiety, and anxiety winds up both parents and babies. If you find yourself being asked these questions in the early days of parenthood, try not to let them stress you out. Instead, emphasize the normality of variation and defuse the tendency for competitive parenting.

While seeking and accepting help is an important component of surviving the first year of parenting, it is also important to set boundaries when necessary, and to remind yourself that you need practical support to care for your baby your way, not advice on how to do things differently. Alloparents should be following your way of handling your baby's sleep, not imposing their own. You do not have to follow their advice or feel anxious about their insensitive questions.

Another area in which you might find yourself receiving unwanted and unsolicited advice is feeding and sleeping—specifically breastfeeding—and we will unpack more about this relationship in the next chapter.

5. Hungry is the night

My typical memories of nighttime feeds are of them merging into one another in a blur, unaware of the day, or the time, and conscious only of a small warm body squirming around next to mine, trying to find a breast in the darkness. The one night feed I do remember clearly happened at the end of August 1997, when my youngest daughter was nearly seven months old. My maternity leave was coming to an end, and she had begun the transition to spending daytimes at a nursery. We had only just started spending half-days apart, and daytime breastfeeding was haphazard, which meant we were feeding frequently at night to make up. Some nights, between 1 and 2 a.m., if my husband was also awake, he would turn on the TV in the bedroom for half an hour. And so it was that the feeding in the early hours of August 31, 1997 was one I will always remember, for when he turned on the TV Princess Diana's car had just crashed in the Pont de l'Alma underpass, and so we were glued to the TV for the rest of the night, hoping for the best and fearing the worst.

I have lost count of the number of times I have been invited to speak at practitioner conferences and study days about the relationship between feeding and sleeping. It is a topic that is always in demand, and if the past thirty years of studying parent–baby sleep behavior have taught me one fundamental thing, it is that for mothers and babies feeding and sleeping are inextricably intertwined—both in how they affect mother–baby nighttime behavior, and in how parent–baby sleep and nighttime care are popularly understood (at least in Western societies).

In the UK, for instance, breastfeeding has been widely considered the root cause of sleep disruption for both babies and parents, and is a common reason given by families for ceasing breastfeeding sooner than they had intended. It is also a key factor in why mothers often bed-share (or "breast-sleep") with their babies (as I did). In places where public health "safer sleep" messaging recommends against all bed-sharing, this creates tensions for many families in their feeding and sleeping decisions. We will explore variations in safer sleep guidance and the reasons for this in detail in later chapters; here, there is a lot to discuss when it comes to feeding and sleeping, and much of it can be contradictory. Let's begin at the very beginning.

Understanding breastfeeding

As we know, the defining characteristic of mammals is our ability to produce and secrete from our bodies a fluid (milk) with nutritional and immunological properties that can feed our babies and keep them alive post-birth. Milk production was a key adaptation in the evolution of mammals, as it allows species to buffer their young from the effects of fluctuations in food availability. Lactation therefore gives mammals a competitive advantage over species that are unable to produce food for their young, and ultimately helped mammals to colonize all habitable ecosystems.

The evolutionary biology of milk production has resulted in the females of each species of mammal producing milk for their offspring that is uniquely constituted in terms of nutrients, reflecting the environmental and behavioral conditions in which it is supplied and consumed.[1] In cases where maternal presence is unpredictable and the opportunity for suckling is potentially short, natural selection has produced milk that ensures infants grow rapidly and thereby survive. For hooded seals the nursing period may be as brief as a week due to the breakup of the ice floes upon which females give birth; female hooded seals produce copious milk that is high in protein and fat, containing up to 200 calories an ounce, allowing seal pups to grow by up to 23kg (50lb) a day, and giving them a chance of survival should they be separated from their mothers.[2] In contrast, primate infants, who are born with the ability to cling, are rarely separated from their mothers and nurse for many months, often suckling several times an hour, receiving diluted milk that is 88 percent water, high in sugar but with relatively low levels of protein and fat. The dramatic contrast between the milk of primates and hooded seals illustrates that mammal milk—including human milk—is not just "milk"; it is a carefully calibrated nutritional substance that has evolved to meet the specific infant survival needs of all species that produce it.

Humans, as a primate species, benefit from the biological consequences of primate lactation—the high sugar content of human milk supports the massive and rapid brain growth that is characteristic of the human baby's first year; the presence of antibodies and immunoglobulins supports immunology and fights infections; while a complex combination of macro- and micronutrients and hormones supports the unique trajectories of human growth and development. Human milk is uniquely suited to the needs of human babies.[3] But before we produce "mature" milk, in the early postnatal period mothers produce **colostrum**, which, although scant in volume (~50ml or 1.7oz on Day 1 postpartum), is important in conferring passive immunity and reducing a baby's exposure to infections, making the early initiation of breastfeeding particularly beneficial to newborns. Growth factors in colostrum, for instance, stimulate the maturation of gastric epithelial cells (cells lining the inside of the stomach), which facilitate nutrient absorption and the development of a physical barrier to pathogens.[4]

At birth, babies' stomachs are tiny and need to receive only a few milliliters of colostrum at every feed. The size of a baby's stomach at different timepoints over the first month is often represented in diagrams using small fruit/nuts to help parents visualize the volume of milk their baby will likely ingest (Figure 5.1). Although as new mothers we are often anxious that we are not producing sufficient milk to meet our babies' needs, it is reassuring to know that only very small quantities are needed in these early days. Most women (unless there are retained placental fragments in the uterus, or other physiological complications) find their milk "comes in" (i.e., they develop a copious milk supply) two to four days after giving birth, when prolactin production reaches a critical threshold to trigger the start of full milk production. I can clearly recall my own first experience of this three days after my first daughter was born; with little warning my boobs were suddenly twice their normal size, rock-hard, and felt like they were on fire! I vividly remember lying on my bed with bags of frozen peas piled across my chest, trying to reduce the pain of that first vigorous surge of milk production.

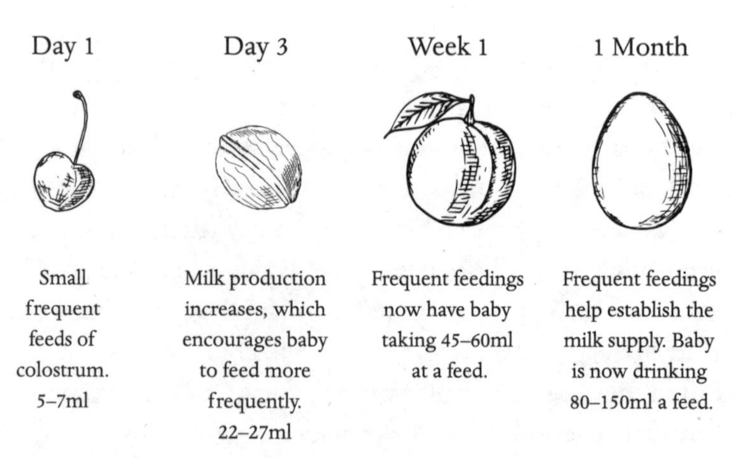

Figure 5.1 Newborn stomach capacity[5]

When a newborn is being fed with formula it is important to remember how *little* newborn babies need to ingest, and to consider how to feed a baby in a way that reflects the breastfeeding experience as much as possible. While some babies go straight to the breast in the hour after birth and suckle vigorously, other babies can be more exhausted from labor or affected by labor analgesics,[6] and mothers who intend to breastfeed might find themselves giving their newborns drops of colostrum on teaspoons or via syringes for the first few feeds until adequate feeding at the breast is established. However, formula that is intended for newborn consumption is typically provided in 60 to 90ml (2 to 3fl oz) bottles, which can lead new parents to think this is the amount their newborn should consume per feed. It is tempting to encourage babies to take the whole bottle, as is sometimes observed in the days following birth,[7] but this is not how newborn babies are designed to feed. As well as the volume of milk they ingest, the way in which babies are given bottle-feeds matters too.

Useful tip

If you are breastfeeding, your baby will receive colostrum for the first few days until your milk supply ramps up. The amount of colostrum a baby needs at each feed in the first few days is tiny, so don't worry if each feed is short, but keep offering the breast frequently. The more frequently your baby stimulates the nipple by suckling, the quicker your milk will come in. If your baby is sleepy after birth (often the case after birth interventions), lots of close contact and frequent opportunities to feed can help, but the process may take longer. Breastfed babies typically lose some of their birth weight during the first week after birth, but they are born with a layer of fat that helps sustain them during this time. If you are feeding formula, remember that very small and frequent feeds are what your baby is expecting, so resist the temptation to have them empty the bottle at every feed. Stop feeding when your baby signals they have had enough, and ask your midwife to explain to you about paced bottle-feeding (see page 105) if you are not familiar with this.

When my brother was born in the early 1970s, breastfeeding rates in the UK were at their lowest, and although my mother had breastfed me for three months in the early '60s, my sister and brother (born four and 10 years later) were both bottle-fed from birth with formula. When babies are fed using a bottle there is a temptation to lean or lie the baby back and almost pour the milk into their mouth; I certainly remember feeding my baby brother this way. If he stopped swallowing to take a break, we would jiggle the bottle teat so more milk ran into his mouth. Of course, the same scenario can happen when babies are fed with human milk that has been expressed and is fed to a baby using a bottle. A baby's usual response in this situation is to keep swallowing so they don't choke!

A slow flow teat on a bottle (i.e., one with a small hole) makes the baby work harder to extract the milk, but this doesn't involve a great deal of effort—mainly compressing the teat between the tongue and palate so the milk squirts out of the hole. If the bottle is tipped at a steep angle, gravity will cause the teat to remain constantly full. To help babies have a bit more control over how much they consume from a bottle, and how fast they consume it, paced bottle-feeding is now recommended, which involves holding a baby in a more upright position and keeping the bottle almost horizontal, so the teat doesn't automatically refill after every suck and swallow.[8] This gives babies the opportunity to stop feeding periodically, and to control how much they consume. But we knew nothing of this in the '70s, and photos of my brother show a chubby baby with hints of having been "overfed" in the plump rolls of flesh on his arms and legs.

In contrast, as I learned when I had my daughters, when newborn babies feed at the breast they must work to extract the milk. Although my letdown reflex would sometimes be forceful and initially squirt milk into my baby's mouth, this was only momentary.[9] Then a baby must coordinate their tongue movements to move the milk from the breast to the mouth, and then to swallow. Breastfeeding is therefore tiring for babies in comparison to formula-feeding, and breastfed babies commonly fall asleep at the breast. In fact, breastfeeding is soporific for both mothers and babies—the action of breastfeeding hormones oxytocin and prolactin cause drowsiness for both members of the dyad—while breastfeeding at night also conveys maternally produced melatonin to babies, increasing the chance they will fall asleep while feeding.[10]

Yet, despite the soporific effects of breastfeeding, popular wisdom is still often heard declaring that giving babies formula is a proven method for encouraging them to: a) sleep; b) sleep longer; and c) sleep through the night. So, let's look at the evidence produced in recent years about the relationship between mode of feeding and mother–baby sleep outcomes.

Feeding and sleeping in the first six months—the subjective view

As we saw in Chapter 4, sleep during the first six months of life is hugely variable as babies are beginning to develop their circadian rhythm and starting to exhibit sleep consolidation (sleeping more at nighttime and less during the day), according to their own individual trajectory. Illnesses and accomplishing various developmental milestones also reduce the predictability and increase the variability of baby sleep. After weeks of sleep disruption parents may begin to wonder whether different feeding choices might help their baby sleep "better" or longer, or disturb them less.

It is likely that the notion that feeding babies formula helps them sleep "better" was grounded in experiential evidence of previous decades—after all, baby formula was frequently adulterated with heavy and indigestible substances such as cereal or baby rice to keep babies satiated (or even alcohol and laudanum in earlier eras, to keep them quiet).[11] Also, as discussed previously, it is easy to "overfeed" a baby when using a bottle, and a "big bottle" of formula before bedtime was (and in some cases still is) a tradition in many families to make sure babies didn't "wake up hungry" during the night. So, it was unsurprising twenty-odd years ago, when we analyzed interviews with 248 parents in the northeast of England, to find a very consistent story about the relationship of feeding and sleeping.

In brief, formula was considered the key to a "good night's sleep" while breastfeeding condemned mothers to months of sleep disruption. Many of the women we spoke to who had ceased breastfeeding during the first three months felt that for them nighttime breastfeeding had been too disruptive, and that their baby disturbed them less at night when they switched to using formula.[12] A consistent theme was that parents were unprepared for the frequency of feeds a breastfed baby needs at night, and they were unwilling or unable to tolerate the sleep disruption this involved. Comments recorded in our interview notes included: "Baby was too demanding and feeding too often. Breastfeeding didn't allow a good night's sleep"; "Baby was too demanding, waking too frequently. Baby now sleeps solid 12 hours at night [on formula]"; "Baby was unsettled on the breast and not sleeping. Now [on formula] baby not fed at night"; "Breastfeeding was too tiring; wanted Dad to help at night."

In the same study, to get a more detailed picture of these experiences, we asked parents to keep sleep logs for their babies over a one-week period during their first and third months, which we collected when we visited for interviews. The parent-recorded sleep logs for breastfed and formula-fed babies showed remarkably different sleep–wake patterns, with the frequency of night-waking differing significantly by feeding type at both time points. Although the reported frequency of feeding at night was the same at one and three months for breastfed babies, there was a significant reduction in night-feeding frequency reported for those fed with formula. While the duration of waking differed little, it seems that the sleep fragmentation associated with breastfeeding led some mothers to switch to formula and to stop breastfeeding, either at night or completely (Figure 5.2).

Our findings were not unique—other research studies had also found that formula-fed babies and their mothers experienced less sleep disruption than mothers and babies who breastfed.[13] So perhaps there is something about formula that means babies wake less often and feed less frequently. Parents are told that breastfeeding is best for babies, but are these studies telling us that—during the night at least—that might not be the case?

Things are not so straightforward. Professor Rosemary Horne

of Monash University in Australia, who is a specialist in infant physiology, explored this question with a study looking at whether feed type impacted the **arousability** of babies (how easy it was for them to wake from sleep). Using polysomnography (measurement of brain waves during sleep), Horne and her colleagues studied 43 healthy term babies at two to four weeks, two to three months, and five to six months. During daytime sleep bouts, repeated attempts were made to arouse each baby using jets of air blown against their nostrils with different amounts of air pressure. Typically, babies are more arousable when in Active than in Quiet sleep, and in this study, when the babies were in Quiet sleep (as identified by the polysomnography traces), there was no difference in the amount of air pressure needed to cause both breastfed and formula-fed babies to arouse. But when they were in Active sleep, breastfed babies aroused more easily (i.e., with significantly lower air pressure in the jets) than did formula-fed babies at two to three months. The researchers concluded that

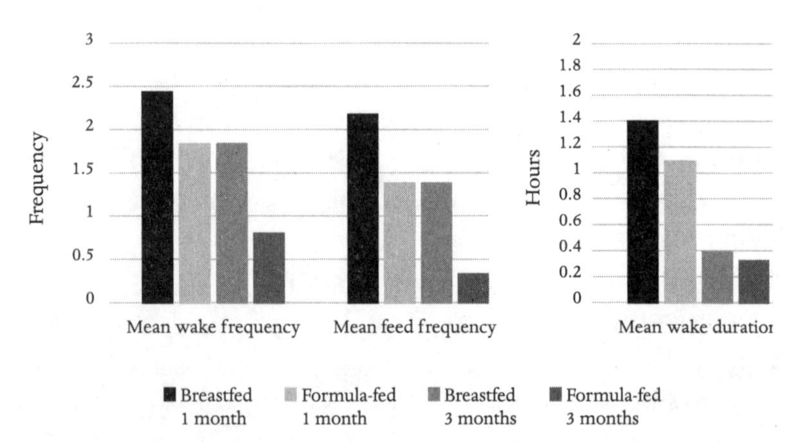

Figure 5.2 Frequency of waking and feeding by feed type at one and three months as reported by parents

breastfed babies have greater arousability from Active sleep at two to three months of age compared with formula-fed babies.[14]

It is unclear whether the phenomenon observed by Horne (a lower arousal threshold for breastfed babies at two to three months) is the same phenomenon that parents were reporting in our interview and sleep log study, but it could be a partial explanation. Further explanation may be found in the high concentration of protein (caseins) found in cow's milk, which may be the cause of more prolonged sleep (or higher arousal threshold) in formula-fed babies, as these are slow to break down in a baby's digestive system, requiring diversion of energy to the gut from the brain while the baby sleeps.[15] In comparison, human milk protein contains much more whey relative to caseins, which babies digest quickly, waking to feed again after a short period.

Twenty years after we conducted the abovementioned research, Alanna Rudzik's "Sleeping Like a Baby" study, also in the northeast of England, found the belief that "breastfeeding means no sleep" was still prevalent.[16] Focus group participants commented: "With breastfeeding you don't know how much they're actually having...if they're hungry they could wake up like two hours later or something," and "Formula and sleep is the key. Breastfeeding and sleep is not happening." But interestingly, while some mothers in Alanna's focus groups held strong opinions that introducing formula was key to promoting baby sleep, another narrative was emerging, with some mothers now challenging the dominant wisdom when they heard it: "I think it's quite an old-fashioned notion that they need formula to sleep better...my mother-in-law and my auntie, who are of that older generation, they're like, 'He's not sleeping through, you need a bottle. You need to give him formula.' Formula and solids. I was told that at three months! [laughs] I was like 'No, I don't think he does.'"

Interestingly, mothers in the focus groups who held the more "traditional view" of feeding and sleeping also expressed firm views that babies could and should sleep in a way that reflected the sleep of the rest of the family. They used the term "routine" to describe this idea, and emphasized the importance of routine for babies, such as: "I've always had all of them in a routine. I believe that a baby fits round your routine, you don't fit around theirs." In contrast, other focus group participants emphasized the importance of prioritizing their baby's sleep patterns, for example, "[Babies] sleep when they need it and forget it. You've got to work round them. And that's all there is to it.... As often as she wakes is when she wakes." [17]

These focus groups showed us how the nature of baby sleep was understood differently by mothers, and this included its relationship to a feeding method. Generally, mothers who were breastfeeding viewed the fragmentary nature of their babies' sleep as expectable and something they had to find ways to cope with while mothers who were primarily formula-feeding felt that their babies' sleep was problematic, and they had to find ways to fix it. The strategies and approaches used to support and promote sleep in each group were aligned with these underlying beliefs about how baby sleep works. The "traditional" group advocated methods where parents take control, such as **cry-it-out**: "I was getting no sleep whatsoever so after six weeks... I asked me mum what she done with us... and she says like do the tough love thing, so I tried it and I just stuck it out and after two weeks she just slept all night."

While it seems very early to impose a cry-it-out approach on a baby of six weeks, this mom followed the advice of her own mother, and it produced the outcome she desired (at least in the short term). In contrast, breastfeeding mothers in the focus groups attempted to align their babies' needs with their own by bringing the baby into bed: "If he's having a night where he wants to nurse a lot I'll put him in bed with me and I'll just sleep and he just latches on when he wants to and it doesn't really interrupt my sleep a great deal."

Mothers' perceptions of the nature of infant sleep and how it relates to a feeding method clearly impact baby-care practices in the first year of life. Among our research participants who wanted to be in control of their babies' sleep patterns, formula-feeding and sleep interventions were preferred; in contrast, for participants who wanted to be responsive to their babies' needs, breastfeeding and bed-sharing were favored. (And of course mothers for whom breastfeeding proves to not be possible can use expressed human milk or formula in a similarly responsive way.) Both approaches have their critics, and each will horrify those who have strong reactions to extinction methods and/or bed-sharing. Those who sit somewhere between these different camps (e.g., breastfeeding without bed-sharing or managing infant sleep without formula use) may struggle the most. What is important to stress is that no single approach to babies' sleep in the early weeks and months will suit everyone, but exploring what is known about the pros and cons of bed-sharing versus sleep training is important for making informed choices.

Feeding and sleeping in the first six months—objective data

Perhaps some of the beliefs about the relationship between formula-feeding and good sleep are familiar to you—from advice you've been given or from reports from friends. And while these self-reported, subjective studies are fascinating for the cultural expectations and beliefs they reveal, researchers are now beginning to accumulate more objective data on the impact of feeding choice on nighttime disruption.

It is not just in the UK that formula supplementation—even of predominantly breastfed babies—is a popular practice, especially at bedtime. There is evidence that within two days after birth approximately 25 percent of breastfed babies in the U.S. are supplemented with formula, with the proportion increasing to 37 percent and 44 percent by three months and six months, respectively.[18] Many times this supplementation is suggested by hospital staff, to allow women exhausted by labor and delivery the chance to rest in the post-birth period,[19] cementing the relationship between formula and sleep from the very start. But despite the widespread use of formula supplementation, it is only relatively recently that research has examined objectively whether this practice—known by many as combination feeding—increases mother or baby sleep time, or reduces sleep fragmentation.

Over the last 10 to 15 years, studies by various research teams have looked at the relationship between feeding and sleeping in multiple settings using objective ways of measuring mothers' and babies' sleep duration, such as **actigraphy** (quantifying sleep patterns using motion sensors) and **video-somnography** (quantifying sleep patterns using video). These studies have repeatedly dispelled the notion that babies fed with cow's-milk formula (at least those fed with the kinds of formula available in the twenty-first century) are "better sleepers" than babies fed with human milk. For instance, in a 2015 UK-based video-somnography study, Professor Ian St James-Roberts and colleagues found that 25 percent of a sample of 100 babies were able to resettle themselves after night-waking at 5 weeks, and 45% were able to sleep for a minimum of five hours continuously at three months of age. Breastfed babies were equally likely to be in the group who did (66%) and did not (63%) sleep for five or more hours and/or resettle themselves during the night.[20] This suggests that formula use is not the underlying cause of babies' sleep consolidation or

self-settling as is often claimed. Why, then, do the mothers of formula-fed babies believe their sleep is better?

Using research studies published between 2012 and 2022, a 2023 systematic review (a comprehensive assessment of every paper published on a topic in a given time period) mapped the relationship between feeding method and total sleep time, number of nocturnal awakenings, duration of awakenings after sleep onset of mothers and babies, and sleep quality of mothers.[21] Most of the 35 studies reviewed found that breastfed babies and their mothers woke up more often at night than those using formula. But the results also showed that there was no difference in total sleep time, or time spent awake during the night, by feed type. Whether babies were breastfed or formula-fed, the amount of time they spent asleep and awake was the same. There was also no difference found in maternal sleep quality by feed type. Sleep quality is a subjective assessment of how well rested you feel in the morning; in the studies reviewed here, sleep quality was captured using validated questionnaires, or questions, diaries or scales created by the researchers. It seems somewhat surprising that while breastfed babies and breastfeeding mothers experience more frequent night-waking in the early months, they do *not* experience less sleep overall in comparison to those feeding with formula, or report poorer sleep quality. One explanation for this is that breastfeeding happens more frequently but for shorter periods during the night, and both mother and baby return to sleep more quickly in comparison with formula-feeding (which may involve waking fully to get up and make the formula); hormones oxytocin and prolactin, which are both released during breastfeeding, cause relaxation and promote drowsiness. Another explanation centers around the presence of melatonin (which triggers sleep onset) in human milk, which is also passed from mother to baby during night feeds, as there is a peak in melatonin concentration in mothers' milk around 3 a.m.[22]

The authors of this systematic review acknowledged some difficulties in comparing the studies they examined due to variations in the ages of babies in the reviewed studies (which covered from birth to 12 months), and variations in the definitions of the feeding types reported. For example, in different studies "breastfeeding" might mean that babies only received human milk (no formula or solids), or sometimes received human milk (with some formula or solids), were only fed directly at the breast, or were included as "breastfed" if fed with expressed human milk. They also noted the issue previously discussed of whether mother–baby sleep data were self-reported or obtained using objective methods. While the impact of the first two issues can be assessed by comparing the outcomes of the individual studies included in the review, the potential effects of parental bias when reporting their own or their baby's sleep are more difficult to unpack. However, several research teams have attempted to do just that. It is worth us considering these studies in some detail in order to understand what we do and don't actually know about feeding and sleeping.

Dr. Therese Doan and her collaborators at the University of California in San Francisco wanted to understand the duration and quality of mothers' sleep in the first month postpartum. At this time babies have not yet developed a day–night rhythm and their very small stomachs mean they need to feed often. They compared the sleep of women who exclusively breastfed at night to those who used formula (and who may or may not have also breastfed) in an ethnically diverse, predominantly low-income group of 120 first-time mothers.[23] Data were generated using actigraphy at one month postpartum. While there were no differences in daytime sleep duration or sleep fragmentation, Doan and her colleagues found that exclusively breastfeeding mothers got on average 30 minutes more night sleep one month after giving birth than mothers who were exclusively formula-feeding (which is a statistically significant difference). When compared to the last trimester of pregnancy, exclusively formula-feeding women experienced 62 minutes less sleep one month after giving birth; exclusively breastfeeding mothers experienced 21 minutes less sleep. Exclusively breastfeeding mothers therefore fared better in objective measures of postpartum sleep. The authors concluded that women should be advised that choosing to formula-feed their baby does not equate with better sleep (regardless of the claims of formula companies—my comment).[24]

But what happens to the relationship between feeding and sleep after the initial transition to motherhood? Does the same relationship between feed type and maternal sleep continue as babies grow and their sleep fluctuates? Dr. Hawley Montgomery-Downs and colleagues studied sleep in 80 women from two to 12 weeks postpartum grouped by feeding method, in this case specifying breastfeeding, formula-feeding and mixed-feeding. The aim of the study was to explore the sleep outcomes of these three groups every two weeks, again using objective measures (actigraphy).[25] This study sample included all mothers, not only first-timers. Montgomery-Downs found that there were no differences in total sleep, sleep efficiency or sleep fragmentation between mothers who were breastfeeding, mothers who were formula-feeding, and mothers who were using a combination of both feeding methods. And although the mothers' reports of their sleep experiences (subjective outcomes) showed more variability across the three feeding categories, these variations were not large enough to be statistically meaningful.

The bottom line from these studies is that switching from breastfeeding to formula offers no measurable benefit to maternal sleep. Even introducing formula at bedtime while continuing to breastfeed at other times offers no measurable benefit—the amount of sleep obtained is pretty much the same. So why is there such a strong public perception that feeding formula will help mothers get more sleep? Before we decide that previous generations of mothers and grandmothers were deluded in their perceptions, or consider what other factors might explain these findings, we should take a look at how feed type affects baby sleep, so we have a complete picture. If the way in which we feed our babies has no measurable impact on mothers' sleep during the first few months of their babies' lives, how does it affect babies themselves? Do mothers have an accurate perception of their babies' nighttime sleep?

Do we really know how our babies sleep?

This question was something I and my colleagues were intrigued by. To find out, Dr. Alanna Rudzik recruited new mothers and their babies who breastfed or formula-fed exclusively, and compared actigraphy and maternal reports of sleep duration every two weeks until each baby was 18 weeks old.[26] What we were looking for was whether mothers' assessments of how long their babies slept differed by feed type, and how closely they matched objective measures. What we discovered was surprising.

We observed that babies' total nighttime sleep duration (all sleep bouts added together) did not differ by feed type. Over the 16-week study, the total sleep increased from an average of 8 hours to 10 hours for both groups while their longest sleep bout remained consistent at between two and three hours. Both groups of mothers reported their babies' sleep duration accurately in the early weeks, but—and here's where things get intriguing—from when babies were 8 weeks old, mothers in the formula group reported that their babies slept around 40–60 minutes more than they actually did (e.g., 10.2 hours vs. 9.3 hours at 12 weeks), while breastfeeding mothers' reports were more accurate (e.g., 9.6 vs 9.2 hours at 12 weeks). But, even more dramatically (Figure 5.3), although babies' longest sleep bout did not differ by feed type, mothers in both groups substantially overestimated their babies' longest sleep period beginning from 10 weeks of age, but did so differently. Mothers of formula-fed babies consistently reported their babies' longest sleep bouts to be three times longer than they actually were (e.g., 7.5 hours reported by mothers vs. 2.4 hours reported by actigraphy at 14 weeks). Exclusively breastfeeding mothers also reported inaccurately but consistently overestimated by lesser amounts (e.g., 5.7 hours vs. 2.4 hours).

So, what is going on here? The picture from the two studies on the sleep duration of mothers (Montgomery-Downs) and babies (Rudzik) is that sleep does not differ by feed type during the first four to five months for either mothers or babies—but that mothers' perceptions of their babies' sleep differ, sometimes dramatically! Figure 5.3 shows that by six weeks of age both exclusively breastfeeding and exclusively formula-feeding mothers in our sample overestimated the duration of their babies' longest sleep period compared with actigraphy, but that by 10 weeks the mothers using formula overestimated their babies' longest sleep periods considerably more than those mothers who were breastfeeding.

That mothers overestimate the duration of their babies' longest sleep bout can be explained by recognizing that we are generally not very good at estimating the passage of time while we are asleep, and all mothers miss some occasions when their baby arouses during the night. But the extreme overestimates that were reported for formula-fed babies—often three times longer than the duration recorded by actigraphy—needs more explanation. There are several, non-mutually exclusive, reasons.

The first is that *where* babies sleep confounds parents' reports of feeding type and sleep. The longest sleep bouts recorded by mothers occurred when babies slept in a room separate from their parents in comparison to when they slept in the same room. Actigraphy data did not vary by babies' sleep location. Not surprisingly, then, mothers have greater awareness of their babies' sleep patterns when they sleep closer together. This is intertwined with feed type because breastfed babies are more likely to sleep in or next to their mothers' beds while a greater proportion of formula-fed babies sleep in a separate room or are moved to one during the first few months.[27]

The second reason, as we have previously seen, is that sharing nighttime feedings with their partner is a key reason mothers give for choosing to feed their babies with formula,[28] and research has found that fathers' involvement in nighttime care is associated with increased maternal sleep.[29] This may mean that some or all mothers in the formula-feeding group who shared night care with their partner had an incomplete picture of their babies' sleep and therefore overestimated sleep time and underestimated night-waking in their sleep logs. But, given the reports of greater sleep disturbance for some formula-feeding mothers in the Montgomery-Downs study, this explanation may only be relevant for a subgroup of mothers with partners who actively contribute to nighttime baby care.

A third reason for mothers' differing perceptions of infant sleep duration by feed type involves the physiological effect of breastfeeding. The sensation of milk buildup in the breasts between feeds can prompt mothers to arouse from sleep prior to their baby waking, and so they may already be awake when their baby wakes to feed. Some studies have also investigated how breastfeeding (or not doing so) is associated with maternal brain response to infant stimuli, reporting that exclusively breastfeeding mothers show greater brain activation responses to their

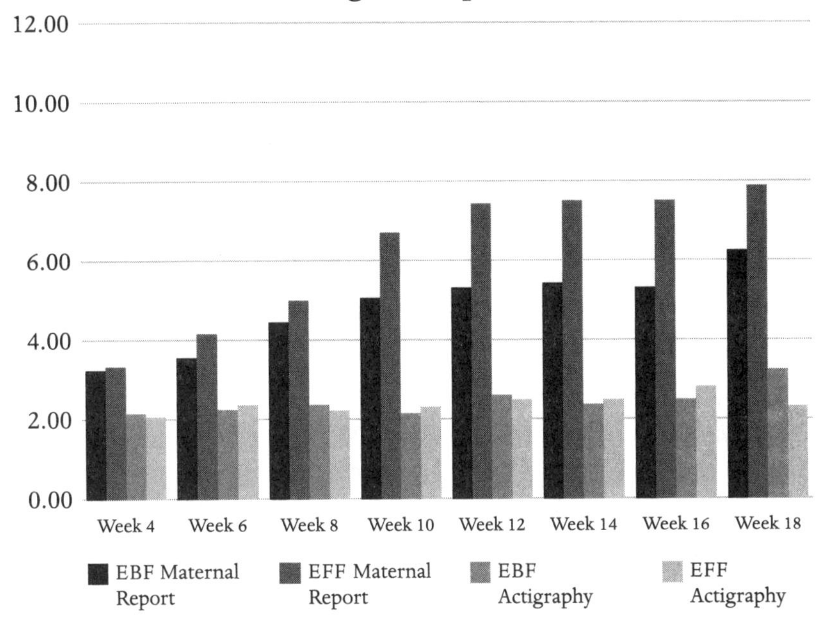

Figure 5.3 Average longest sleep bout for exclusively breastfed and formula-fed babies (EBF = Exclusively Breastfed; EFF = Exclusively Formula-Fed; Black columns = maternal report (sleep logs); Gray columns = actigraphy)

baby in comparison with exclusively formula-feeding mothers.[30] Lactation-related arousals or brain activations may potentially underpin greater awareness of baby sleep patterns among breastfeeding mothers.

Does all of this mean that the popular perceptions about formula-feeding, breastfeeding and sleep that we previously described are founded on fantasy? Were our mothers and grandmothers deluded? No, I don't think they were. I think a combination of factors coalesced to present them with a convincing picture that formula-fed babies slept "better." In previous decades the composition of formula milk for babies was quite different from today. Nowadays, large cow's-milk protein molecules that are difficult for babies to digest are hydrolyzed, homogenized and chemically modified in various ways to break them down into smaller, more digestible components, as formula manufacturers continue to try to create a product that is like human milk. It is very likely that earlier versions of formula did indeed cause babies to sleep for longer periods while their bodies attempted to digest a kind of milk they did not have the gastrointestinal tools to process. On top of that, babies commonly slept in separate rooms from their parents, where they were less likely to be heard.

Useful tip

If you begin your journey into parenthood with the intention that your baby will be breastfed, it is almost certain that someone somewhere along the line will advise you that this means your baby will never sleep, and recommend introducing formula to avoid this, or to improve your sleep. You are now empowered to respond that although parents often feel their baby sleeps better when they introduce formula, studies show that this is not the case, and that breastfeeding mothers and babies obtain as much if not more sleep overall than formula-feeders. While you may wake more frequently to breastfeed, you will spend less time awake and return to sleep more quickly. And if you choose to bed-share, you don't even have to get out of bed!

Nowadays there is little to be gained in terms of sleep for either mothers or babies from switching between human milk and formula milk in the first few months of a baby's life; the only clear benefit is for sharing nighttime feeds, and this can be done using expressed human milk. While there are many reasons why you may feed your baby with formula, the evidence we now have shows that getting more sleep will not be one of them.

Feeding and sleeping after six months of age

What about the rest of your baby's first year? Does how we feed our babies after they are six months old—the age at which it is now recommended to introduce solids—influence sleep during later infancy?

Unfortunately, there are few studies that have used actigraphy to assess the sleep of mothers and babies by feed type after six months, so we have to rely on studies based on parental reports, with all the lack of accuracy this entails.

Dr. Amy Brown and Vicky Harries from Swansea University explored how feed type affected sleep outcomes for older infants in a 2015 study involving 715 UK mothers and their six- to twelve-month-old babies (mean age 35 weeks).[31] Mothers reported on their baby's typical night-waking and night feeds alongside any breastfeeding and the frequency of solid meals. They found that 79 percent of the babies in the study regularly woke at least once a night, with 61 percent receiving one or more milk feeds—breast or formula—at night. The good news was that both night-waking and night feeds decreased with age, and again no differences in night-waking or night feeding were reported for mothers who were breastfeeding or formula-feeding. And despite what some might say about giving babies solids earlier to improve nighttime sleep, the study found no association between age of introduction to solids and night-waking—babies who received more milk or solid food during the day were less likely to feed at night, but they were not less likely to wake (according to mothers' reports).

The authors concluded that it is common for breastfed babies to wake and feed during the night in the second six months postpartum. And although breastfed babies in this study were reported to be fed more frequently during the night than were formula-fed babies, they were not reported to wake more—formula-fed babies also continued to wake but were not fed (although without actigraphy or video-somnography, the frequency of waking cannot be confirmed).

This picture was reiterated by a 2024 study in Norway examining breastfeeding and sleeping patterns in six-to-twelve-month-old breastfed infants.[32] Researchers received data from 342 mothers who reported their babies slept for 11 hours per night (median duration) with 97 percent waking at least once per night, and 94 percent being breastfed at least once per night. The authors found that only 17 percent of babies in the study fell asleep without parental assistance, and that 47 percent of the breastfed infants fell asleep while breastfeeding. The other babies fell asleep while being bottle-fed, rocked, held or cuddled, or with the presence of a parent in the room. There was some variation by age in how long the babies slept: babies who were 9–12 months slept on average 30 minutes less per night than those ages 6–8 months. Babies ages 6–8 months woke on average three times (median), with a range of 0–15 wakes; in comparison, at 9–12 months the night-wake frequency was four (median) with a range of 0–15. Nighttime breastfeeding was common across both age groups—the median nighttime breastfeeding frequency was three, with a range of 0–15 in the younger group and 0–8 in the older group.

Curiously, babies who were more frequently breastfed at night slept longer than those who were less frequently breastfed. As noted with younger infants, this may be a function of where babies slept, as bed-sharing is related to frequent night-feeding and to longer sleep duration. Presumably, if your mother is right next to you when you wake up, it does not take long to latch on, feed a bit, and fall back to sleep, but if she is in another room and you have to wake her to come and get you, the whole process will take longer and the amount of time you are asleep will be shorter, especially if you have to go back to sleep by yourself in your crib. The potential downside for mothers is that although breastfeeding is easy during bed-sharing, babies tend to wake up and feed back to sleep more frequently (presumably because you are right there, and they can). But as they also sleep more than when you breastfeed but don't bed-share, the decision as to which scenario is preferable is yours.

So, night-waking and night breastfeeding are common behaviors for babies who are breastfed throughout the second half of the first year of life, despite babies also consuming other foods during this period. These studies challenge the suggestion that complementary foods will help babies sleep through the night, and do not support the notion that babies are waking due to hunger—rather, the Norwegian study suggests that after six months of age babies are breastfed because they wake, not that they wake so they can breastfeed. Although it is often said that babies no longer need to breastfeed at night once they are over six months old and are consuming solid food, this is based on a narrow nutritive view of the breastfeeding relationship that assumes the nutrients obtained from breastfeeding are now being obtained from other food. But if your baby is (for whatever reason) not consuming enough during the day, night feeds are still an important component of their diet. Furthermore, as we saw in Chapter 1, obtaining contact with and comfort from their mother's body is an important aspect of the mother–baby relationship, and babies' need for the comfort of breastfeeding to help them return to sleep quickly has not been outgrown at six months. For mothers and babies, breastfeeding is an efficient way to return to sleep quickly and obtain more sleep overall, and is often facilitated by bed-sharing.

Useful tip

If you continue to breastfeed your baby past the six-month mark, it is likely you will hear from someone that doing so provides your baby no nutritional value once they are consuming solids, and particularly so if you breastfeed your toddler past their first birthday. You may even be told in derogatory tones that you are allowing your baby to "use you as a pacifier." For many babies, breast milk continues to provide calories and nutrients while they practice eating solid food, and they continue to benefit from all of the immunological properties of breast milk for as long as they continue to receive it. But it is also important to remember that the breastfeeding relationship between a mother–baby dyad is about much more than the transfer of milk or the effects of its components. The ability of breastfeeding to support emotional regulation and restore equilibrium is extremely important: the physiological effects of breastfeeding hormones calm and relax you both, help you sleep, resolve distress and provide comfort. Let's reframe "being used as a pacifier" as "using your superpower" to help your child regulate their emotions and support their well-being.

Key things to remember about the feed–sleep relationship

As you now know, the composition of human milk means that babies digest it quickly and wake frequently to feed throughout the day and night when breastfeeding is their primary sustenance. Lactating mothers need their babies to feed frequently day and night in order to sustain their milk supply (milk has to be removed for more to be produced). In contrast, the cow's-milk formula available for babies in previous decades was difficult to digest, meaning formula-fed babies would wake and feed less frequently than their breastfeeding counterparts, with no detrimental effects on the sustainability of their food source.

It is easy to see how comparing the sleep of breastfed and formula-fed babies in past decades fueled popular perceptions about infant night-waking and how to encourage early settling. But as recent studies show, there is no longer any difference in the sleep duration between breastfed and formula-fed babies or their mothers, even though mothers may still report differences in their sleep experiences. It is time we challenge out-of-date notions about feeding and sleep when we encounter them, and redefine popular understanding of the feed–sleep relationship.

The most likely reasons why we (in general, because there are always exceptions) might perceive that formula-fed babies sleep more than breastfed babies, when objective sleep studies find no difference, are: a) because we may miss some of our babies' night-wakes when the sharing of nighttime care is working effectively; b) because the biology of lactation affects our sleep and awareness; and c) there are differences in sleep proximity that influence our awareness, with breastfeeders more likely than formula-feeders to bed-share.

The relationship between feeding and sleep location, particularly bed-sharing and breastfeeding, will be unpacked in the next two chapters. Where breastfed babies sleep, and how safety issues are addressed, are important topics we now need to explore.

6. A bed of one's own?

When we were pregnant with our first child, my husband and I looked at cots (or cribs, as we were in the U.S.) in the local department stores and discovered them to greatly exceed our budget, so we decided we would build the wooden sleeping furniture our baby needed. My husband's grandfather had a carpentry workshop in his basement, and having purchased wood at the local lumberyard, we spent several weekends handcrafting mortice and tenon joints, sanding, gluing and staining to create a basic but sturdy and relatively attractive-looking baby cage. As things turned out, the crib was barely used by our first child, and so when we moved to the UK it was transported with all our other belongings in a shipping container to our new home where it was barely used by our second child. After accompanying us on two further house moves and following a long spell in the rafters of our garage, we finally consigned it to a Dumpster 20 years after building it. It ended up being barely used because our babies bed-shared habitually from birth, and then intermittently from around 18 months after moving into their own beds and bedrooms.

Despite our crib being barely used, it is important to note that all babies do need a crib or other safe space where they can be parked on those occasions when a parent is required to attend to something else and cannot hold—or keep their eyes on—the baby, and no one else is available to hold them. It is not safe to leave a baby unattended on an adult bed, sofa, armchair, etc., and so some form of baby cage is needed for safety.[1]

I decided that we would bed-share toward the end of my first pregnancy after contemplating the realities of breastfeeding at night. Our accommodation was small—a double bed barely fit in our bedroom, and there was no space for the crib we had painstakingly crafted. The only place for it was in another room down the hall. I tried to imagine what it would be like getting up multiple times a night, collecting the baby, going to the living room or back to bed to feed, then returning them down the hall after feeding, only to repeat the process a couple of hours later. I had read about bed-sharing and wondered whether it was the answer, so I phoned a friend—a senior academic I had gotten to know while doing my PhD research in Puerto Rico. She had a small child, and I trusted her judgment. "Would you tell me about how you and [son] managed nighttime breastfeeding and your sleeping arrangements?" I asked her. "Sure," she said. "[Husband] and I just had [son] sleep in bed with us. It was so much easier to breastfeed that way than having him in a crib, and we all got so much more sleep." "I've been wondering about bed-sharing," I told her. "So you think it's an OK thing to do?" I asked. "Yes," she replied, "it worked amazingly well for us, he still sleeps with us now." That decided it: we would bed-share.

And so, from the day they were born, both of my daughters slept all night every night at my side—the first began in hospital where we spent two nights, the second at home where we returned three hours after delivery. Even though they were sometimes sick all over me, even though they sometimes kicked me in the face, even though we sometimes had to change the sheets at 3 a.m., I can say with complete honesty that sleeping with my babies was one of the best decisions I ever made.

Studying bed-sharing

When I began studying parent–baby sleep in 1995 I was most curious about bed-sharing, but the topic left some of my colleagues bemused. "How will you study that here? No one in the UK does it," one of them asserted. As by this time I was the mother of a three-year-old, I knew many families that had or did share a bed—but as my colleague illustrated, to the majority of the UK population, bed-sharing with babies was invisible.[2]

Despite the fact that babies have slept in their mothers' arms for millennia, and indeed this is where the majority of the world's babies still sleep every night, in the UK (as in the U.S.) not only was bed-sharing stigmatized, it was practiced covertly. This had been the case since the spread of Freudian insights into early childhood experiences and the complex dynamics of family relationships had reached parents and shaped parenting practices via Dr. Spock's *Common Sense Book of Baby and Child Care* in the post–World War II era. By the end of the twentieth century when it captured my interest, parents still did it, but they lied about it—to one another, to their families, and to their health professionals. Consequently, many parents who were bed-sharing with their babies (regardless of whether they were doing so openly) felt criticized and chastised while others were simply too afraid to do it. Yet within those families where it was commonplace, it was viewed as practical, normal and commonsense. I wanted to lift the veil of stigma that was draped over the topic of bed-sharing and explain to the critics and the uninformed why bed-sharing with babies was important for many families, and why expectant parents needed to know about it, to have opportunities to discuss it with others, and to learn about its benefits, hazards and nuances.[3]

Biological anthropologist Dr. James McKenna from Pomona College, California (and later professor of anthropology at University of Notre Dame), had been studying parent–baby bed-sharing in the U.S. since the early 1990s in collaboration with sleep scientist Dr. Sarah Mosko at the University of California, Irvine's Sleep Disorders Laboratory. It was reading an article about their research during my first pregnancy that captured my attention.[4] Jim was interested in the regulatory effects of mothers' bodies on babies during sleep, and especially **sleep synchrony** in breastfeeding dyads. In an influential project he and Sarah Mosko conducted overnight studies of 35 breastfeeding pairs sleeping together and apart using video and polysomnography of both mothers and babies to understand how sleep architecture was influenced by each other's presence or absence. The study was revealing about nighttime feeding patterns, finding that nighttime breastfeeding was twice as frequent for those mother–baby pairs who regularly bed-shared (every 97 minutes on average) than for those who normally slept separately (feeding every 187 minutes on average).[5] But even more important was what the study showed about the *way* babies slept when they were next to their mothers. They found that when they were bed-sharing, babies experienced more lighter (Active) sleep, less deep (Quiet) sleep, and longer total sleep time (sleep duration) than when sleeping alone. As we've seen, Active sleep is when babies' brains are growing, making new neural connections and processing information, and also when they are most easily aroused.

McKenna and Mosko also found that both babies and mothers experienced more overlapping arousals, waking up within moments of each other and promoting synchrony in their sleep cycles.[6] Just like their babies, bed-sharing mothers also experienced more light and REM sleep and less deep (non-REM) sleep, but for mothers there was no difference in overall sleep duration. Sleep contact provides babies and mothers with a demonstrably different sleep experience than solitary sleep, where bed-sharing mothers are more attuned to their babies during the night, are less likely to miss their babies' cues, and have heightened awareness of their presence. This is important to bear in mind when we think about bed-sharing safety, as we will in Chapter 7. While many mothers are nervous to try bed-sharing because of concerns about safety, McKenna proposed that the solitary sleeping baby's experience of prolonged deep sleep with fewer arousals may in fact increase their vulnerability to the phenomenon known as **Sudden Infant Death Syndrome** (SIDS), when babies die unexpectedly and without explanation during sleep. He noted that breastfeeding and bed-sharing (which he later labeled **breast-sleeping**) mothers were particularly responsive to their babies during the night.[7] These comparative studies provided the foundation of a scientific evidence base about bed-sharing against which epidemiological and psychological assumptions could be tested, and soon more researchers began to build upon this foundation.

In Bristol, Peter Fleming (professor of infant health and developmental physiology at the University of Bristol) and then-PhD student Jeanine Young (now professor of midwifery at the University of the Sunshine Coast in Queensland, Australia) set up a temporary mother–baby sleep lab where they recorded overnight video and physiology from 10 mothers and their babies who alternately slept in the same room and the same bed for two nights each month over a five-month period.[8] Their findings were consistent with those of McKenna and Mosko: during bed-sharing, mother–baby sleep states had greater synchrony, and significantly more interaction was observed, than during room-sharing (crib by bed). When bed-sharing, mothers aroused and responded quickly to their babies, touching and breastfeeding them more frequently than when the babies were in a crib by the bed. Babies were warmer when bed-sharing, were able to adequately regulate their core temperature, and did not overheat.[9] These early lab studies of bed-sharing clearly show that the sleep of both mothers and babies is altered by sleeping together and sleeping apart. It is worth noting again that separating mothers and babies for sleep was one of the biggest unacknowledged experiments in human behavior of the twentieth century.

The helplessness of human babies, their need for contact and for frequent nighttime feeding, makes mother–baby bed-sharing a predictable human behavior, and indeed it is common practice in many areas of the world. However, in some countries—such as the United States—a mother's arms are considered the *least* safe place for a baby to sleep, with mother–baby bed-sharing considered inappropriate, inadvisable and dangerous. We will delve into the reasons for this in the next chapter, but first we need to take a closer look at why, when and how parents and babies sleep together—and what we know about the pros and cons of bed-sharing. As with many other baby sleep topics, the evidence is rarely clear-cut and heavily influenced by prevailing cultural attitudes.

How common is bed-sharing?

My journey to explore bed-sharing began in 1995 in the north-east of England in collaboration with my then-PhD student Elaine Hooker, talking to 60 families (half of which were having their first baby) attending antenatal classes at a local hospital. We were curious to learn about parents' intentions and subsequent practices with their babies at night, and were unsurprised to find that very few (only four) first-time parents had any intentions of bed-sharing before their baby's birth; most gave reasons for not doing so, such as "creating bad habits," "spoiling the baby," the importance of fostering independence, and fears about overlying—all common themes in popular discourse related to bed-sharing. In contrast, all of the expectant couples who already had a child acknowledged that bed-sharing was likely. Despite most first-time parents declaring they would never bed-share, when we asked if they imagined ever bringing their baby into bed only five couples were adamant this would never happen—the majority anticipated doing so if their baby was ill, for breastfeeding, and to help their baby go to sleep, but all said they would return their baby to a crib before they fell asleep themselves (which reflected the guidance of the mid-1990s).[10]

Three months after their babies were born, 70 percent of the first-time parents had bed-shared with their baby at least occasionally. Of these, two babies were sleeping all night every night in their parents' bed, half were sleeping in their parents' bed for part of every night, and a handful slept in their parents' bed occasionally. Most of the babies regularly sleeping in their parents' bed were breastfed. Yet most of these parents did not consider themselves to be "bed-sharing"—their baby had a crib they were supposed to sleep in, and this was where their babies generally began the night, and so this was their babies' reported sleep location, regardless of how little time they actually spent there. This was our first glimpse of how much unacknowledged parent–baby bed-sharing was happening in the UK, especially among breastfeeding families. The cultural ideology against bed-sharing was so powerful that even parents who regularly bed-shared rationalized that they weren't really "bed-sharers"—they just brought their baby into bed to feed, and sleep with them for a bit of the night, or half the night, or longer.

This discovery was important for several reasons. It confirmed that bed-sharing was not irrelevant to families in the UK as was believed by pediatricians and others. It illustrated that parents who were adamant they would never bed-share found themselves doing so. And it revealed that as parents we not only do things covertly that we think might be criticized by others, but we also delude ourselves that we are not actually doing them—we rationalize that what we are doing is somehow different. Consequently, studies have underestimated the prevalence of bed-sharing when researchers have accepted parents' answers at face value rather than probing about all the places babies sleep. These issues convinced me that parent–baby bed-sharing was something we needed to understand better, and talk about more, especially given the mounting evidence that some forms of bed-sharing (or its alternatives, like sofa-sharing) could be dangerous for babies. Then as now, I felt strongly that parents needed information to be able to make informed choices.

In the late 1990s, with a growing research team, I explored what happened at night in homes with new babies by collecting data from over 250 families in a northern English town.[11] Over two one-week periods when their babies were one and three months old, parents kept sleep logs of when and where their babies slept, and then were interviewed. The data revealed that 54 percent of the babies bed-shared (which we defined, based on our previous study, as when a baby slept in bed with an adult who was also sleeping, for any part of the night) at least once during the two weeks when sleep logs were recorded, and the interviews found that 70 percent had bed-shared at some point in the three-month period. Most babies began bed-sharing in the first few weeks of life. We categorized "habitual bed-sharing" as when a baby slept in their parents' bed all night every night; "combination bed-sharing" as when a baby slept in a combination of locations, bed-sharing for part-nights on most nights; "occasional bed-sharing" as once a week or less; and "never bed-sharing" as babies whose parents reported they had never slept with an adult. Two-thirds of those who slept in their parents' bed were exclusively or partially breastfed, the largest group being "combination bed-sharers." In comparison, just over a quarter of babies fed with formula bed-shared, and these were evenly split between combination and occasional bed-sharing (Figure 6.1).

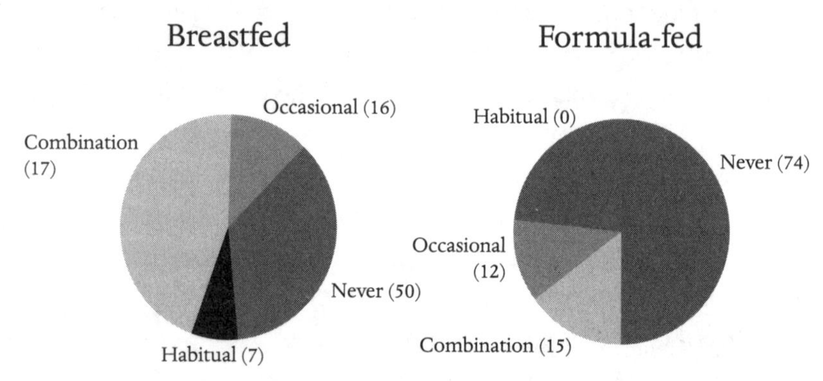

Figure 6.1 Bed-sharing frequency for breastfed and formula-fed babies[12]

When I spoke at conferences about how many families were bed-sharing, other researchers (often older male statisticians and pediatricians) were incredulous. They claimed there must be something unusual about our study sample—they felt the findings must be inaccurate because they contradicted their assumptions. Fortunately, Dr. Pete Blair, statistician for the CESDI study,[13] a large case control study of Sudden Infant Deaths in England and Wales, had data on sleep locations for over 1,000 control babies from five different health regions of the UK that allowed us to test this claim. Using the same measures, we compared the CESDI data with our local northeast England data and found they were identical. This gave me confidence that our data were accurate: around half of all UK families with babies bed-shared to some extent in their first three months.[14] Other studies conducted during the surrounding decade (1998–2008) in a wide range of Western locations—including Canada, New Zealand, Australia and the U.S.—all produced similar figures for bed-sharing prevalence, confirming that, contrary to popular perceptions, bed-sharing with babies was a common practice in many Western societies (Figure 6.2).[15]

Our initial studies around the turn of the millennium found that in the UK, bed-sharing was widespread (although under-acknowledged), strongly associated with breastfeeding, and not strongly related to lower socioeconomic status, as had been widely believed. This picture was different from what was being reported in the U.S. and New Zealand at the time, where bed-sharing was characterized as a baby-care practice confined to culturally distinct and socioeconomically deprived minority communities. However, it is now clear that bed-sharing is both prevalent, and widespread, across cultures and societies.

Why do many of us bed-share with our babies?

In many parts of the world the straightforward answer to the question of why we bed-share with our babies is, simply, because it is the customary thing to do. Bed-sharing is the way that babies sleep in most African, Asian, South American and Central American countries, including wealthy postindustrial nations such as Japan and South Korea. Bed-sharing is also reported to be common in multiple European countries, such as Spain, Italy, Norway, and Sweden. But in most Western societies, because bed-sharing has not been considered "normal" for the past 80 years or so, we seem to need some further justification. In research interviews parents have explained that the most common reason for

Sample	Proportion bed-sharing	Data collection method	Reference
6,268 NZ families	43%	Interviewed at clinics	Tuohy et al. 1998
410 U.S. families	46%	Questionnaires	Gibson et al. 2000
44 Australian families	46%	Questionnaires	Rigda et al. 2000
253 NE UK families	47%	Interviews/ diaries	Ball 2002
394 U.S. families	48%	Interviews	Brenner et al. 2003
8,453 U.S. families	47%	NISPS telephone survey	Willinger et al. 2003
210 NL families	40%	Questionnaires	Van Sleuwen et al. 2003
1,095 UK families	48%	HV interview	Blair & Ball 2004
12,290 UK families	49%	Postal survey	Bolling et al. 2007
2,300 U.S. mothers	42%	Questionnaires	Hauck et al. 2008
293 Canadian families	72%	Questionnaires	Ateah & Hamelin 2008

Figure 6.2 Bed-sharing prevalence estimates in Western countries

bringing their baby into bed was for the ease and convenience of nighttime breastfeeding. Parents who were unprepared for the frequency with which breastfed babies need to feed, particularly in the early months, reported that their baby's frequent feeding and their own need for more sleep were reasons for stopping breastfeeding, but those participants who were committed to continued breastfeeding—and those with experience of previous children—had used bed-sharing to ameliorate the impact of frequent nighttime feeds. Breastfeeding mothers often commented that when bed-sharing they barely needed to wake up in order to let their baby feed, a finding that has since been replicated in many studies in the UK and elsewhere,[16] and one which certainly resonates with my own experience. Where bed-sharing is not related to breastfeeding, families may use it as a way of settling a baby who is unhappy, irritable or occasionally unwell.

While breastfeeding, settling and illness were the three primary motivations prompting our UK study participants to bed-share, some parents who were working during the daytime explained that bed-sharing made breastfeeding possible when they resumed work (the night-feeding helping to maintain milk supply), while for others, including several fathers, it was a pleasurable opportunity to reunite with their baby from whom they were separated during the daytime. For a couple of families we interviewed, bed-sharing was not a matter of choice but of circumstance; due to lack of funds or facilities, these young parents found themselves sleeping with their baby because there was no alternative, and in one case all three family members were sharing a single bed in temporary accommodations.[17] In contrast, some families had intentionally bought as large a bed as possible so that all family members could sleep together. For these parents a family bed meant habitually sleeping with the youngest family members, and allowing older children to come and go between their own beds and the family bed as they wished. Other researchers have since documented many of the same bed-sharing motives in other Western countries.[18]

The wide array of explanations from parents confirm that bed-sharing is a varied activity, intentionally implemented for numerous reasons under a range of circumstances while also happening unintentionally and without planning, and out of necessity rather than choice, in others. Perhaps you might be thinking of bed-sharing or are doing so already, or maybe you are questioning whether it can be done safely, or whether you should mention it to a new parent you know as a way to cope with frequent feeding or sleep disruption. So, having gained a sense of parents' reasons for bed-sharing with their baby, let's now have a look at the ways in which we go about implementing it.

How do we do it?

Serendipitously, my second daughter was born just as our bed-sharing research at Durham was gaining momentum, providing the perfect opportunity for Elaine and I to work out how to film overnight videos of bed-sharing families in their homes. As McKenna and Mosko's polysomnography study and Fleming and Young's video study both took place in hospital sleep labs, we were keen to observe naturalistic bed-sharing behavior. So, during the spring of 1997, my daughter and I, and my long-suffering husband, became the first guinea pigs for in-home parent–baby video-somnography. Elaine and I spent much of my maternity leave trialing the placement of tripods, cameras, video recorders and infrared lights around the bedrooms of my family's small semidetached house in Durham to work out how we might solve the problems of filming in the dark, for eight consecutive hours, from fixed vantage points while keeping the baby in view, allowing parents to start and stop the recordings whenever they wanted, without creating an obstacle course around the bedroom, and of course, doing it all on a shoestring budget.

After lots of trial and error we devised a system that worked well enough and began recruiting for volunteers to be filmed sleeping with their babies. A university press release for the local newspapers was picked up by the regional morning TV news channels, who of course wanted some video clips to illustrate the story—which is how footage of my husband, baby and me all snoozing together became the "human interest story" on a breakfast episode of *Look North*, much to the amusement of our friends and neighbors. Thankfully, the media exposure led to sufficient volunteers, and Elaine trekked around the northeast of England for several months installing video equipment in bedrooms, and later disassembling it and retrieving videotapes. We then began the long process of coding and analyzing the footage, minute by minute, creating massive spreadsheets on which each family's data were summarized. As time went on, the available equipment became smaller and more sophisticated, and with various research grants we were able to move from using video recorders and long-play VHS tapes that we carried around in cardboard boxes with cumbersome tripods and infrared lights, to custom-built equipment cases containing camcorders and CD-writers, and eventually to low-lux digital cameras and laptops with automated software for behavioral data analysis. Despite the technological improvements over time, some of our most enduring and important research outcomes were produced using equipment that we had MacGyvered[19] in my bedroom with my family as guinea pigs.

The evidence of *how* breastfeeding mothers sleep with their babies was the most important information to emerge from these pioneering studies. I remember my first talk on this topic to the pediatric department of the hospital where we had previously recruited participants during their postnatal stay. I described how breastfeeding mothers appeared to instinctively sleep with their babies in a very specific way, lying on their side with their baby next to them, the baby positioned on their back with their head at their mother's breast level. Without any instruction, mothers curled up around their babies, with their knees under the baby's feet and their arm outstretched or bent above the baby's head, creating a space with their bodies for the baby to sleep in (Figure 6.3), which we called the "C-position," and others labeled the "cuddle-curl."

During the night, babies leaned toward their mothers to feed, either staying on their side for a while or returning to a **supine** (on the back) position. While sleeping, mothers roused, monitored their baby's temperature and breathing by touching the forehead and placing a hand on the chest, readjusted the covers, then resumed sleep. Usually, they were unaware of having done this until we showed them their video. I knew, of course, that I also slept in this exact same way with both of my babies, but what happened at the end of this talk still took me by surprise.

A woman I didn't know was sitting near the front of the auditorium, and as I finished speaking, she immediately raised her hand. She introduced herself as one of the hospital pediatricians. "We have never met, and you don't know me at all," she began, "but you have just described me precisely. Everything you said is exactly how I slept with my baby, and I had no idea that other mothers did the same—I thought it was just me!" This experience was repeated many times over the next 25 years as women who heard me speak recognized themselves in the videos of the mothers we filmed as we attempted to capture naturalistic bed-sharing behavior in domestic settings.

The characteristic sleep position we documented for breastsleeping mothers and babies was reinforced by later observations of other research teams,[20] and our own observations of mothers' and babies' first night on the hospital postnatal ward, where first-time mothers who were randomly allocated to sleep with their baby in their bed spontaneously adopted this position without instruction.[21] Although this behavior evolved in a very different sleep context than Western domestic bedrooms or hospital post-natal wards, the mother's instinct to protect her baby is reflected in her behavior, and has been described as follows:

> When mothers curl up around their infants for sleep they construct a space in which their infant can sleep constrained by their own body, protected from potentially dangerous environmental factors—be they predators, cold weather, or the suffocation hazards of quilts and pillows. In the current Western context, therefore, bed-sharing breastfeeding infants sleep flat on their mother's mattress, away from pillows, in a lateral or supine position. Despite the fears of coroners and pathologists that infants may be overlain, when a breastfeeding mother sleeps curled up around her infant in this way she cannot roll forwards onto it, and neither can any other co-bed-sharers lie on the infant without lying on the mother also.[22]

It is likely, then, that breastfeeding mothers may avoid or reduce the potential hazards associated with babies sleeping in

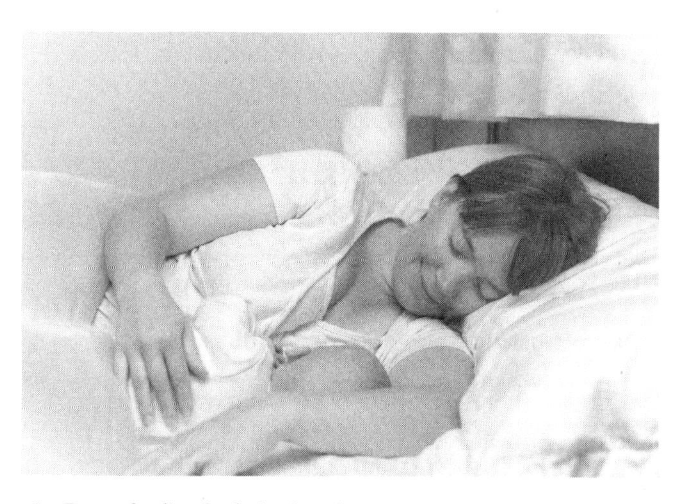

Figure 6.3 Breastfeeding bed-sharing sleep position (aka breast-sleeping), courtesy Rob Mank Photography

adult beds, such as suffocation and overlaying, due to this characteristic behavior. This interpretation was reinforced when we observed notable differences in bed-sharing behavior of some parents who had never breastfed.[23] Our videos showed that some bed-sharing formula-fed babies were placed level with their parents' faces rather than at breast or chest height, meaning these babies were positioned on or between their parents' pillows, while breastfed babies were positioned flat on the mattress away from any pillows. Mothers who had never breastfed spent a smaller proportion of sleep time facing their baby and did not adopt the protective sleep position with the same consistency as mothers who breastfed. Never-breastfeeding pairs experienced fewer arousals during sleep, as well as significantly fewer synchronous arousals. These differences in the sleep behavior of breastfeeding and non-breastfeeding mothers and babies during shared sleep are consistent with descriptions of the effects of breastfeeding hormones in promoting close contact between mothers and babies, including heightened responsiveness and awareness,[24] and suggest that breastfeeding and formula-feeding may create experientially different contexts for bed-sharing.

Useful tips

Make your bed as safe as possible for your baby, even if you think you will never bed-share, just in case. Also see Chapter 7 for when bed-sharing should be avoided.

- Check that there are no gaps between the bed and furniture or walls that your baby could slip into. Move the bed away from the wall or tightly pack the gaps.

- If you have a hard floor, think about lowering the height of your bed in case your baby falls off. Do not place cushions as a "landing area"; they are a suffocation hazard if your baby lands on them face down.
- Remove all heavy bedding and use lightweight layers that will stay put at your waist height. Wear a long-sleeved shirt or cardigan if you need extra warmth.
- Remove any unnecessary cushions and pillows from the bed.
- Position your baby on their back on the flat mattress, with their head below the level of the pillows.
- Lie on your side facing them, positioning your arm above their head, preventing them from pushing themselves up the bed into or under your pillow. Position your bent knees under their feet, preventing them from wriggling down the bed or under your covers.
- Dress your baby in layers appropriate for the room temperature, such as an undershirt and a sleeping bag.
- Avoid having other children sleeping next to the baby and avoid having pets on the bed.
- If you place your baby between you and your partner, ensure your partner knows the baby is in the bed, and baby is close to you.
- Once your baby is independently mobile, double-check for gaps around the bed, including the headboard and footboard.

Breastfeeding promotes bed-sharing, which supports breastfeeding

During those exciting and frustrating days of extra-long-play VHS tapes, mothers who forgot to turn the video recorder on, and fathers who helpfully "adjusted" the cameras after we had carefully positioned them, we added a new dimension to parent–baby sleep research, not just in documenting aspects of infant sleep and nighttime care that had been previously neglected, but also in imagining the possibilities for new questions that could be explored using this approach. At yet another conference I recall chatting with a neonatologist (one of those amazing doctors who take care of very premature babies). We were talking about whether bed-sharing improved breastfeeding outcomes and how this could be studied. I remarked that we'd need to randomize moms and babies to different sleep conditions to compare breastfeeding outcomes, but that this would be impossible to do in a domestic setting as you can't expect a family to stick to an assigned sleep arrangement in their own home. "I wonder..." I mused, "whether we'd get permission to randomly allocate moms and babies to different sleep conditions during their postnatal hospital stay?" (which in the early to mid-2000s in the UK was two to three nights for straightforward vaginal deliveries for first-time moms). "Ahhh," said my colleague—who unbeknownst to me had oversight of his hospital's postnatal wards—"I think we might be able to help with that!" Which is how, a couple of years later (because setting up studies and getting funding for them is a slow process), we found ourselves making overnight videos of mothers and their newborn babies on the postnatal ward of a big teaching hospital in the north of England. This project (which we have already touched on) aimed to find out whether facilitating prolonged physical contact (e.g., by bed-sharing between mothers and babies) in the early postnatal period would help with breastfeeding initiation. Before we delve into this study more deeply, however, we need to know how newborn babies breastfeed and learn a bit more about the biology of lactation.

It is widely recommended that immediately after birth mothers and babies should experience up to an hour of uninterrupted skin-to-skin contact before they are transferred together to the postnatal ward, due to the important benefits for both mothers and babies.[25] During this hour (as we have seen) a healthy, vaginally delivered baby will move through Widström's nine stages of behavior,[26] culminating in the first breastfeed and a period of sleep, a manifestation of the newborn baby's survival instinct to find the breast and start suckling without assistance.[27] This instinctive behavior has been documented in multiple postnatal settings spanning Sweden, the U.S., Egypt and Uganda. The importance of uninterrupted skin-to-skin contact in the immediate postnatal period is hugely important for the initiation of breastfeeding. But what, we wondered, happens after this initial hour? If you just "do skin-to-skin" for an hour or so after delivery, is it sufficient? What happens next?

In most maternity facilities, after transfer from the delivery suite, mother–baby proximity involves **rooming-in**, with the baby at the mother's bedside in a see-through bassinet that resembles a fish tank. In some countries this may happen only during the daytime, with the baby removed to a communal nursery at night, but elsewhere (including in all UK postnatal wards, and in **WHO/Unicef Baby Friendly Initiative** accredited hospitals worldwide) 24-hour rooming-in is the norm, with mothers performing all aspects of their baby's care. Research into the benefits of rooming-in has shown that removal of babies at night to neonatal nurseries results in less frequent breastfeeding and a greater likelihood of breastfeeding failure.[28] Contrary to the popular belief that mothers sleep better during the immediate postpartum if their babies are cared for by staff, studies have found that nighttime mother–baby separation does not result in an increase in either quantity or quality of maternal sleep or in maternal alertness the next day, while babies who spend their nights in neonatal nurseries sleep significantly less and cry more than those at their mothers' bedside.[29]

Rooming-in is encouraged, therefore, to foster frequent breastfeeding and ensure mothers feel comfortable handling their babies before they leave the maternity unit. It is assumed that mothers and babies will feed more frequently when rooming-in than when their babies are in a nursery, but we wondered whether a plastic bassinet at their mother's bedside gave babies sufficient opportunity to reinforce their initial hour of delivery-room skin-to-skin contact and allowed them to continue practicing instinctive breastfeeding behavior. Our hypothesis was that facilitating close physical contact via bed-sharing for the entire postnatal hospital stay would allow mothers and babies to engage in more frequent breastfeeding bouts, leading to more successful initiation of breastfeeding, and in turn perhaps supporting breastfeeding duration.

With the help of my late friend Dr. Martin Ward-Platt, the previously mentioned consultant neonatologist, my research assistants and I recruited pregnant women anticipating normal deliveries and intending to breastfeed to take part in a trial. Sixty-one newborns, vaginally delivered with no opiate analgesia (which makes mothers and babies drowsy and affects breastfeeding behavior), were randomly assigned to one of three arrangements for their postnatal stay: 20 mothers "roomed-in" with their baby in a crib at their bedside; 23 bed-shared using a three-sided crib (sidecar crib) attached to their bed; and 18 bed-shared with the baby with a mesh safety rail attached to their bed. Moms and babies were videoed for the first two nights after birth using a night-vision camera remotely controlled by the mothers, and all participants were contacted by telephone at 2, 4, 8 and 16 weeks after birth to ask about the babies' health and feed type.

When we analyzed the overnight videos we found that babies in physical contact with their mothers at night (i.e., those in the bed and sidecar crib) fed more frequently than babies in the separate crib (where mothers and babies were unable to touch each other due to the height and the walls of the crib).[30] We saw multiple instances of babies in cribs making **feeding cues** (mouthing their fists, rocking their heads, clicking their tongues) but giving up when they couldn't find their mom, and of mothers sleeping through their babies' quietly wakeful periods, or encouraging them back to sleep by jiggling the crib frame. In contrast, those babies in the bed and sidecar crib only had to start **rooting** (seeking the nipple by turning their head and nuzzling around), or even squirming, for their mothers to feel them moving and offer the breast. When watching these videos the memories of my first nights with my eldest daughter in our hospital bed in a small-town hospital in Maine came flooding back.

Responding promptly when a baby gives cues that they are ready to feed and practicing frequent suckling in the days and nights right after birth are crucial for triggering a mother's breasts to produce milk: a process that is regulated by the hormone prolactin. Whenever a baby touches the mother's nipple, prolactin released by the mother's brain increases rapidly, with the amount of prolactin being directly related to the intensity of nipple stimulation. More prolactin is produced each time the baby attempts to feed, so frequent attempts are important, especially at night when there is a greater prolactin surge than during daytime.[31] The onset of copious milk production (e.g., when mothers feel their milk "come in") is regulated by the amount of prolactin produced, which is in turn affected by the timing of the first breastfeed, and the frequency of feeding at the breast. When babies feed early and frequently, their mothers produce more milk more quickly than if the first feed is delayed, or if babies are uninterested in nursing thereafter (which may occur following C-sections, or the use of labor analgesia that makes the baby sleepy). In a nutshell, frequent early surges of prolactin speed up and increase milk production, while infrequent suckling is associated with delayed milk production and a less prolific supply.[32]

By understanding that frequent early suckling affects how quickly and strongly mothers' milk appears, you will hopefully grasp how mother–baby sleep contact can affect breastfeeding initiation, and therefore see the relevance of our postnatal ward sleep location trial. Mother–baby sleep contact promotes more frequent nipple stimulation, suckling, and prolactin surges (which are bigger at night), thereby stimulating more rapid milk production (lactation) and a more prolific milk supply.

But there is more to consider, because stimulating prolactin production at the beginning of lactation also influences long-term milk production, and this hinges on the successful development of prolactin receptors in the breast tissue itself. We produce prolactin receptors in our breast tissue during the first three months postpartum, and these receptors are crucial in keeping milk production going when the process of lactation stops being endocrine regulated (controlled by the brain), and autocrine regulation (controlled by the breast) takes over.[33] This means that frequent early feeding, especially at night, supports effective early milk production, *and* supports a sustainable long-term milk supply.

Useful tip

If you feel strongly that you want to breastfeed your baby in the early days, or for a sustained period, talk to your midwife about how you can create an environment that encourages frequent feeding throughout the duration of your hospital stay (night and day).

A common reason reported in the U.S. and UK for stopping breastfeeding is that a woman isn't producing enough milk (or feels as though she isn't) several weeks into her breastfeeding journey.[34] If the development of prolactin receptors in the early breastfeeding period is hindered by infrequent feeding, particularly at night, we wondered whether mother–baby separation at night played a role in reduced milk supply and early breastfeeding cessation.

We hypothesized that mothers and babies in close contact on the postnatal ward (e.g., bed and sidecar crib locations) with unlimited opportunity for frequent early suckling would breastfeed for longer than those in the crib group, where babies fed less frequently during our trial. When we followed up our participants, we discovered that the proportion of babies in the crib group who were exclusively or partially breastfed fell rapidly compared to the bed and sidecar crib groups. Bed-sharing supports breastfeeding initiation but may also support the continuation of breastfeeding (we couldn't be sure of the latter as it was a small video trial, not a large breastfeeding trial). The cultural pressure to get babies to sleep alone from a very early age is clearly at odds with the biology of breastfeeding, and I fear many women who might desperately want to breastfeed yet find themselves struggling don't know this. Following well-meaning advice to "teach" your baby to sleep alone as soon as you come home from the hospital may actually undermine your success in establishing breastfeeding. Rather than warning new parents that lots of nighttime contact and feeding will establish "bad habits," we should be helping parents understand that it will establish sustainable feeding.

Useful tip

Frequent feeding is key for supporting milk production. To help your milk come in, put your baby to the breast frequently day and night. Allow your baby plenty of time and opportunity to practice and work out for themselves how to latch and suckle. Sometimes babies are a bit uncoordinated, and it can take a while for them to figure things out. Make it as easy as possible for both of you by staying in contact, preferably in bed (bed-sharing safely), and recruiting friends and family members to look after you, the house, and the rest of your family until you and your baby have a comfortable feeding pattern established.

To find out whether early sleep contact in the postnatal period influenced breastfeeding duration we needed to do a larger trial with more moms and babies. This time we recruited 1,200 mother–baby pairs who intended to breastfeed, and gave them either a sidecar crib or a separate crib for their postnatal hospital stay. They then reported where their babies slept and how they fed every week for six months. In this trial—known as the NECOT (North-East Cot) trial—we included all babies born via vaginal deliveries, but not C-sections. The overall trial results showed no difference between the two sleeping arrangements for breastfeeding duration.[35] But when we partitioned the sample into those who had uncomplicated and unmedicated births versus those with interventions such as epidurals or assisted delivery, we found that those moms and babies who were given a sidecar crib after an uncomplicated birth breastfed for significantly longer than those who were given a separate crib, reinforcing the results of the video study.[36] But for those mom–baby pairs who had birth interventions, the type of crib received had no effect on breastfeeding duration.

In a follow-up video trial, PhD student Kristin Tully (now research assistant professor in obstetrics and gynecology at the University of North Carolina) compared the use of sidecar cribs and normal bedside cribs on the postnatal ward following C-section delivery. She found no difference in breastfeeding outcomes, which was explained by the challenges all mothers and babies faced with breastfeeding initiation.[37] Post-C-section babies were observed to be very mucousy and sleepy and were much less interested in suckling than the unmedicated vaginally delivered babies we had videoed previously.

When coding the overnight videos, however, Kristin also documented more unsafe infant handling and unsafe bed-sharing (such as mothers sleeping with babies on pillows across their laps) in the group who received the separate crib compared to the group who used the sidecar crib. Reaching into a standard hospital crib at their bedside to retrieve or return their baby was clearly painful and difficult when women had a fresh C-section incision, and this caused them to avoid returning the baby to the crib. In contrast, caregiving was easier and much safer when the baby was located in a sidecar crib.

Our sidecar crib studies therefore found that when birth is straightforward, bed-sharing enables more frequent nighttime feeding, which in turn supports longer breastfeeding. When birth is more complicated, feeding is often disrupted, creating greater breastfeeding challenges that can be overcome by a two-night intervention supporting mom–baby sleep contact on the postnatal ward.[38]

When the moms and babies in the NECOT trial left the hospital, 56 percent bed-shared at home during the first three months (regardless of which trial group they were in). Twice as many of those who bed-shared at home breastfed to six months (or beyond) compared with those that did not bed-share.[39] This again supports the argument that bed-sharing facilitates breastfeeding, but this may also be explained by mothers with a strong commitment to breastfeeding being more likely to choose to bed-share—indeed we found that those mothers who chose to sleep with their babies, and who subsequently breastfed for at least six months, also had the strongest prenatal intentions to breastfeed.[40] Bed-sharing is therefore a successful strategy used by many mothers to help them achieve their goal of breastfeeding to six months or beyond.[41] The larger implication of this is that preventing mother–baby bed-sharing undermines the ability of mothers to achieve their breastfeeding goals.[42] Together these studies show that breastfeeding and bed-sharing are a mutually reinforcing and predictable behavioral complex, and that not only does discouraging bed-sharing undermine breastfeeding, but supporting early bed-sharing protects against later breastfeeding failure.[43]

Key things to remember about bed-sharing

We have seen in this chapter that an evolutionary perspective views the mother–baby dyad as a mutually dependent unit, behaviorally and physiologically intertwined in a multitude of ways. When we are separated from our babies at night in the early postnatal period our ability to lactate and their ability to establish breastfeeding is disrupted more than is commonly acknowledged, and this is just one example of disrupted connections. At the time when I initiated our hospital trials in the mid-2000s, a quarter of UK mothers who began breastfeeding stopped within two weeks, and only a fifth were still breastfeeding at six months,[44] and there were, of course, many reasons for this. But I knew, both from my own experience as a breast-sleeping mother, and from the hundreds of moms and babies in our studies to that point, that keeping moms and babies in close proximity at night in the early postnatal weeks makes breastfeeding initiation and maintenance much easier than it might otherwise be by supporting the fundamental biological links between us and our babies.

Thirty years ago, when I stood up at academic and medical conferences and told elderly male pediatricians that they were undermining efforts to improve breastfeeding in the UK by insisting babies should sleep alone and "learn" to self-settle from an early age, I met plenty of resistance. Changing attitudes about how and where babies sleep can be likened to turning an ocean liner. But it has turned. As we will see in the next chapter, the UK now has a very different approach to bed-sharing than the one I encountered in 1995.

There are a wide range of reasons besides breastfeeding as to why you might choose to bed-share with your baby, though this is the most prevalent one. It is important that all parents are aware of how to bed-share safely, including the positions to adopt and where to place your baby.[45] There has been limited research on fathers' bed-sharing behavior, which is also important to understand in more depth.[46] In the next chapter we will discuss the circumstances in which bed-sharing is inadvisable and why, and also think through how to make the bed-sharing environment as safe as possible for your baby throughout their first year.

Anthropological and evolutionary perspectives have allowed us to ask novel questions about parent–baby sleep, explore nighttime care differently, and better understand variations in baby-care behaviors and how they are implemented. Research informed by anthropology and evolutionary biology has shown that parent–infant bed-sharing serves many different purposes for different people, and if done carefully and with forethought it can be incredibly beneficial, particularly for breastfeeding and coping with sleep disruption. However, it is also well documented that sleeping with a baby can be done in hazardous ways, which is important for us to now explore.

7. Do not go gentle into that good night

(Content warning—chapter discusses infant deaths)

Sadly, in the few months after birth, some babies die unexpectedly during sleep. In wealthy countries these deaths, although infrequent, became noticeable once hygiene, sanitation and healthcare improved and infectious diseases declined. At the end of the nineteenth century, for instance, infant mortality rates in the UK were high, with 150 babies dying of every 1,000 babies born[1] (which was actually much lower than the 300–500 deaths per 1,000 births in preceding centuries), but by the mid-twentieth century this fell to 34 deaths per 1,000 births, few enough that each baby death could be individually investigated. Pathologists reported that some apparently healthy babies were dying inexplicably during sleep (then known as "cot death," later named Sudden Infant Death Syndrome, or SIDS), and studies to investigate potential causes began in the 1960s. After 60 years of work, epidemiologists now know a great deal about how to reduce SIDS, and infant mortality in the UK is at its lowest rate ever (four deaths per 1,000 births), and while some of these are tragic and avoidable sleep-related accidents, in other cases there is no clear explanation or underlying cause for why an apparently healthy baby might die unexpectedly in their sleep.

When my youngest was about 14 months old she began sleeping in her own room for the first half of the night, then coming into our bed to breastfeed in the wee hours. Every night, as many of us do, I checked on her and her older sister before I went to bed. My husband was bemused by this: "They're asleep," he would say. "What's going to happen to them?" But, like many of you, I was anxious about their safety whenever they weren't by my side; my instinct was to check on them, and so I did. One night as I quietly poked my head around my youngest daughter's door, I could hear her making an unusual sound. She was fast asleep, on her back, nothing covering her face, yet she was making this odd little grunt of exertion every few seconds. She was covered with a loose-weave cellular blanket that she'd slept under many times. As I tried to move the blanket to check her over it seemed stuck to something, and I could feel that one of the threads was pulled tight. Gently feeling in the half-light from the doorway, I traced the tight thread from the blanket, over my daughter's left shoulder, around the back of her neck, across her throat, and to her left hand, which was scrunched against her neck. Wrapped tightly around one of her fingers was the end of the loop of thread. Somehow, she had managed to catch her finger in a loop, pull it out of the blanket, and wrap it around her neck as she turned over, to create a ligature across her throat. As she'd pulled on the thread in her sleep, trying to extricate her finger, she'd tightened the string around her neck to the point that it was cutting deeply into her skin.

As I released her finger from the loop, and the tension of the thread around her throat loosened, the grunting noises ceased and she began breathing normally. In bed (after throwing out the blanket), I lay imagining what we might have awoken to find had I not made my routine check.

For the first 12 months, infant sleep safety guidance aims to alert us to the most common unsafe scenarios so we know how to protect our babies at night, but we still need to remain vigilant about unpredictable situations. Understanding the vulnerabilities of babies and the well-known risks they might encounter can help us identify less predictable risks and intervene when necessary.

Research into Sudden Unexpected Death in Infancy (SUDI)

In the UK, around 300 deaths a year happen suddenly and unexpectedly to babies under 12 months old, which is about one in every 2,300 born (3,400 in the U.S., or one in every 1,100 born).[2] Some of these, about 100 per year in the UK, are **sleep-related accidental deaths**, which include suffocation, positional asphyxia and entrapment—while the rest (around 200 a year) have no clear explanation. Together they are called **Sudden Unexpected Death in Infancy** (SUDI in the UK, SUID in Canada, the U.S. and elsewhere), a term covering all unanticipated deaths of babies that were healthy 24 hours previously.[3] If, after a full investigation including the baby's death scene, medical history and postmortem, no clear cause can be ascertained, a death is classified as an unexplained SUDI and is typically referred to as SIDS.[4] This means SIDS is not a cause of death, but a label designating a baby death with no clear cause. SIDS deaths peak between two to four months of age.

Although these numbers can seem incredibly scary to a new parent, the good news is that most SUDI are avoidable. The purpose of infant sleep safety guidance, which in the UK everyone should receive antenatally and postnatally, is to make sure parents know about SUDI/SIDS and how to avoid scenarios where they occur. In the late 1980s, UK SUDI rates were much higher than they are today; in 1988 sudden infant death affected almost 1,600 UK families,[5] prompting high-profile TV and newspaper campaigns.[6] Baby sleep safety guidance brought about a sharp fall in unexplained deaths in all countries where it was introduced.

It is interesting to note, however, that although most parents generally followed sleep safety guidelines, the campaigns had little effect on general attitudes or expectations around baby sleep. This, in my view, was because these campaigns focused closely on instructing parents what to do and what not to do, using simple messages, which worked to reduce deaths. But they did not help parents develop an understanding of babies' biological needs or limited competencies, which with hindsight was a missed opportunity to change *attitudes* toward baby sleep, and not just practices.

In our research we have found that today's new parents have much less awareness of unexpected baby deaths than we did 30 or more years ago, and rarely know anyone who has lost a baby. Yet, as young adults, my friends and I knew of several families who had experienced a "cot death." This means that today, sleep safety guidance not only has to help parents understand what sleep safety risks are but must also raise awareness that the risks are real, without provoking excessive anxiety. It is a tricky business.

On top of this, infant deaths are now a health inequity issue. Safer sleep campaigns reach many families, but not all, and SUDI tends to cluster in our most impoverished communities and in families who are least likely to access antenatal care and most likely to refuse or avoid postnatal home visits. The opportunities to offer SUDI information and support to these families are limited, and new approaches are needed to prevent the remaining preventable baby deaths.[7]

In the U.S., sleep safety campaigns brought about disproportionate reductions in unexpected baby deaths across different communities and strata of society. While SIDS rates plummeted among the white middle classes and well-educated portions of society, those living in poverty, experiencing structural inequalities, and subjected to racism saw more modest reductions in infant deaths.[8] The discrepancies in U.S. parents' abilities to engage with and implement sleep safety guidance over the past 30 years are well documented by Laura Harrison, whose book

Losing Sleep offers a detailed discussion of how messages about infant sleep safety have affected U.S. parents differently according to their social location, have privileged certain types of parenting over others, and stigmatized parents of color in punitive ways while ignoring the overwhelming role of social determinants on infant mortality.[9] Reducing sleep-related deaths equitably across the entire population is the current challenge.

Where does sleep safety information come from?

Initial attempts to reduce unexplained baby deaths were largely based on the circumstances (such as the sleep environments) in which babies died, and the characteristics of those babies (such as gender, age, prematurity), but it was very difficult to identify risks that might be avoided without knowing how these babies, their homes or their care differed from babies who survived. How do you tell what is relevant and what is not? For two decades U.S. researchers observed that most deaths occurred among babies who were placed to sleep in the prone position (chest down), but because U.S. babies generally slept in this position at the time, the observation did not stand out as important.[10] To overcome this difficulty, epidemiologists co-opted a research method from infectious disease investigations that allowed them to compare babies who died (cases) with babies who didn't die (controls) of the same age and from the same location (the **case-control method**). This helps researchers identify how two similar groups differ, pinpoint factors that are more prevalent among the cases than the controls, and assess how big each risk might be.

Of course, risk calculations are only as good as the data on which they are based, so where data are incomplete—questions about baby care are poorly specified, cases and controls aren't well matched, or parents don't provide accurate information—the risks identified can be misleading, biased or overinflated. For this reason, in most areas of health research, the hypotheses that are generated by case-control studies are usually tested using more rigorous methods, such as randomized trials, before health policy or clinical recommendations are produced. With SUDI, however, it is not possible to test the legitimacy of risk factors using randomized trials, as this would mean asking families to agree to be randomly allocated to having their babies sleep in a way that might—if the hypothesis is correct—result in the death of some babies. As this is clearly unethical, the risk factors generated by SUDI case-control studies are used to inform policy and guidance *without* further testing, and so should be used with caution. But as sleep safety messaging aims to be simple and clear, the information presented to parents has tended to be more assertively instructional than cautiously educational. Let's look at some examples.

Sleep position: the key risk factor

The key risk factor to emerge from case-control studies was sleep position. Dozens of studies worldwide confirmed that SIDS cases more often slept on their front (prone) while controls more often slept on their back (supine). This doesn't mean that every baby who sleeps on their front will die, but the chance of it happening is increased.[11] This data gave rise to guidance in the late 1980s (UK) and early '90s (U.S.) to always place babies to sleep on their back, known in many countries as the "Back to Sleep" campaigns.[12] As most babies were previously put down for sleep on their front, the number of infant deaths fell in each location as authorities recommended that parents place babies on their back. Most UK parents readily adopted this change, with prone sleep for babies falling from 89 percent to 24 percent after the UK "Back to Sleep" guidance. Clear, simple advice about sleep position has therefore saved thousands of babies' lives over the past 30 years.

Placing babies on their backs to reduce SUDI is something we've been familiar with ever since, and there are clues as to why it is important. Small babies have very heavy heads, weak necks and poor muscle tone, and when chest down can get their face pressed against the sleep surface, compromising their ability to breathe. Being face down is also linked to babies overheating and rebreathing exhaled carbon dioxide, so there are numerous reasons to avoid it.[13] Placing young babies to sleep on their front on a flat horizontal surface is also not an evolved human caregiving behavior, being uncommon before the mid-twentieth century.

You may worry that your baby will choke while on their back if they vomit or regurgitate milk; however, babies' swallowing and breathing anatomy doesn't work like that of adults, where liquid from the stomach flows into the trachea (windpipe). For babies, the position of the tube to the lungs (trachea) and tube to the stomach (esophagus) are arranged differently. When a baby is supine, the trachea is above the esophagus, so if a baby vomits the fluid runs back into the stomach and not to the lungs.[14] Nevertheless, parents do lie babies on their side due to fear of choking, but this is an unstable position; babies who've died after being put down to sleep on their side have typically been found face down.

As babies age, they begin to change their own sleep position. SIDS primarily affects babies under six months, and older babies who can turn from back to front and back again will find their own sleep position without increased risk, but until they can do this easily it is suggested to return them to their back if they turn onto their front.

Useful tip

When putting a baby down to sleep, doing so on their back, on a flat, horizontal surface, has the lowest risk of SIDS and does not increase the chance of choking. Tilting or inclining the surface on which a baby sleeps is sometimes suggested to avoid reflux, but no studies have shown that this is effective. Giving babies smaller feeds and feeding them in an upright position is more helpful. Inclined sleep surfaces (such as tilted cribs and baby seats) can cause positional asphyxia, as the weight of the baby's head pulls it forward and kinks their windpipe, compromising their breathing.

In the decades that followed the initial studies on sleep position, more case-control studies were completed and new risk factors were found. The evidence for sleep position is very strong, with over 40 studies examining increasingly more precise questions about the position in which the baby was: a) placed for sleep; and b) found.[15] But the strength of the evidence for other risk factors varies depending on how precisely researchers defined the variables they examined, how many cases and controls were affected, and how many studies looked at each issue (and did so in the same way), and so we should consider each risk carefully.

Sleeping alone

Whether day or night, the risk to babies increases if they are alone for sleep, and this risk is substantially reduced when they sleep in the presence of a caregiver.[16] Guidance therefore advises keeping babies in the same room as their caregiver for all sleep for at least the first six months in the UK (or 12 months in the U.S.). This doesn't mean you can't leave the room briefly to go to the bathroom or answer the door, but it does mean not putting the baby upstairs for a nap while you get on with tasks downstairs. It is the presence of an adult caregiver that is protective—both because you are able to physically check on the baby regularly, and because the noise of your activities helps trigger babies' arousal from deep sleep, prompting them to breathe. Arousal is an important protective response in reducing deep sleep and supporting protective airway mechanisms,[17] especially given human babies' neurological immaturity.

Early in my academic career I was invited to give a departmental seminar—an informal talk for staff and postgraduates about our current work. I had not long started studying baby sleep and was contemplating the role of Western beliefs in unexpected infant deaths.[18] With this in mind, I prepared a talk that highlighted some popular ideas about baby sleep that were incongruent with sleep safety. For examples I turned to a pile of parenting manuals that I had collected on my office bookshelf, searching for quotes that depicted British attitudes toward the nighttime care of babies. It did not take long to find what I was looking for: the desirability of fostering independence, self-control and self-reliance, and "teaching" good sleep habits. *The Baby Book* by Dr. Rosemary Sturgess (1977) was a best-selling parenting manual of its time. The quote I found there had a particular poignancy for this topic, and admonished parents whose instincts were to keep their babies close during the nighttime. Dr. Sturgess reinforced the idea that babies should get used to sleeping alone from the night they came home from the maternity hospital, by telling parents: "He's not going to die before the dawn, just because he is alone in there. . . ."

History sadly shows that between the time this quote was published (1977) and my seminar (1997), thousands of babies had, in fact, "died before the dawn" while sleeping in rooms alone—evidence that drives international guidance encouraging parents to sleep in the same room as their babies at night, and to keep babies in the presence of their caregiver for daytime sleep.[19] Tragically, our cultural preference for leaving babies to sleep in a room on their own, together with guidance from clinicians in the 1950s to place babies chest down for sleep, has caused us to care for babies in ways that are incongruent with their biological and developmental capabilities.[20]

Useful tip

It can be helpful to prepare two safe sleep spaces for a baby, one in your room to be used at night, and one in the main living area to be used during the day. A portable sleep space such as a portable bassinet, playpen, Moses basket or baby stroller can be used, so long as it is firm, flat and level, and it is easy for you to see your baby when they are in there. Even if you intend to use a sling or adult-worn baby carrier for your baby during the day, it is helpful to have a safe place prepared for when you might need to lay your baby down.

Smoking

Ensuring babies arouse regularly and are prompted to breathe is relevant to another aspect of infant care that is strongly linked to the prevention of SUDI: keeping babies smoke-free. Exposure to cigarette smoke before and after birth increases the risk of sudden infant death, with at least 40 studies finding up to a five-fold increase in risk.[21] A U.S. study found that smoking more than one cigarette per day doubled the baby's risk of death, likely due to the effect of nicotine on babies' heart rate, blood pressure and arousal. Babies who were smoke-exposed during pregnancy, for instance, have a blunted arousal response and are less able to wake if they encounter a physiological challenge, such as difficulty with breathing. Compared to babies who were not smoke-exposed, they are less likely to gasp for breath when their airways are blocked or covered.[22] Parents and practitioners often ask whether this increased risk of SUDI also applies to e-cigarettes or vaping, but at present there are no case-control studies that include sufficient numbers of babies whose parents vaped to be able to assess the chance of SUDI with vaping. I would suspect, though, that if the vapes contain nicotine (and some vapes include high doses of nicotine), the effects may be similar to those of cigarettes.

Prematurity

Another group of SUDI-vulnerable babies are those born prematurely or with low birth weight (LBW). For these babies, sadly the risk is elevated from birth: the proportion of preterm and LBW babies experiencing SUDI is about four times that of term babies, and is inversely related to gestational age (that is, more SUDIs occur among early than late preterm babies).[23] This is again related to these babies' lower heart rate, blood pressure and reduced arousal compared to those with normal birth weight and full-term gestation. While this information will understandably cause anxiety if you are the parent of a baby who was born prematurely, understanding the need to be extra vigilant about following safer sleep guidance can help you protect your child.

Multiples have also been found to have an increased risk of SIDS, which is attributed to the fact that most twins and higher-order multiples are born prematurely. If you have twins who were born at term, their intrinsic risk is no greater than that for singletons.

Useful tip

Parents of premature or low birth weight babies, and babies who were smoke-exposed in pregnancy, are all encouraged to follow safer sleep guidance closely, given the clear evidence of increased risk of SUDI for these babies. This means placing them on their backs when putting them down to sleep, ensuring this is on a firm, flat, level surface, and keeping them smoke-free postnatally.

Avoid using any tips, techniques or devices to encourage these babies to "sleep deeply," and always keep them with you. Let other caregivers of your baby know they should be vigilant about sleep safety too.

Absence of breastfeeding

Something that has been shown to substantially reduce the risk of sudden infant death is breastfeeding. Multiple studies have found that fewer breastfed babies are SUDI victims, and the most recent analysis shows that babies breastfed for two months or more have a 50 percent lower chance of SIDS than those breastfed for less than two months, with the protection offered by breastfeeding continuing until a baby is at least six months old.[24] Studies examining the sleep of breastfed babies show they have more frequent arousals and a lower arousal threshold (they arouse more easily).[25]

Consuming human milk, specifically tailored for our species, is less physiologically challenging for babies to process than milk produced for the young of a different mammal species that has been industrially modified, or ultra-processed, into food for human babies.[26] But as formula use may be unavoidable, it is important for parents and other caregivers to know it is associated with reduced arousal from sleep and greater SUDI risk, so they can be alert to avoiding other risk factors, including using practices and products that encourage babies to sleep more deeply than normal or for prolonged periods.

Overheating and soft surfaces

Overheating, overwrapping (many layers), sleeping on soft surfaces, and having soft items in the sleep environment have all been found more often in SUDI cases than control babies.[27] However, some studies have looked at the number of layers on the baby, some room temperature, and some babies' skin temperature to assess overheating, so exactly what to avoid is unclear. Studies have found up to 28 percent of SIDS cases had their heads covered, and 69 percent of suffocations were attributed to soft bedding.[28]

Useful tip

Because of the risks of overheating and suffocation, parents and caregivers are cautioned to keep soft, squishy items that can insulate a baby's head or block their airways out of their sleep space, including loose blankets, duvets, pillows, crib bumpers, cushioned products and soft toys. This also includes removing hats indoors, as babies need to lose heat from their heads to cool down.

In those countries where sleep safety guidance is issued, then, parents are informed that babies are safest on their backs for sleep, in a clear flat, level space, with no overheating or suffocation hazards present. In the UK the phrase "feet to foot" is sometimes used, which means placing the baby's feet to the foot of the crib, and is suggested when parents cover their baby using well-secured sheets or blankets tucked firmly under the mattress. This "feet to foot" guidance was common before baby sleeping bags became popular, as placing a baby's feet at the bottom of a crib stops them from wriggling under the bedclothes and getting their head covered.

In the early 2000s I was asked by TAMBA (the UK Twin and Multiple Birth Association, now the Twins Trust) to explore how sleep safety guidance was implemented by parents with twins or multiples, and whether there were any specific issues they should advise twins' parents about. We surveyed TAMBA members about their baby sleep practices, and parents were particularly interested in whether (and how) they could co-bed their twins in the same crib. Many families had insufficient space for two cribs in the parents' bedroom, and when their babies outgrew Moses baskets at three to four months they either had to move them to a different room, or co-bed them in a single crib to keep them close at night.[29] We videoed twins sleeping together and apart at home and monitored their physiology in our sleep lab.[30] The only problem we identified with co-bedding in a full-size crib was if loose bedding was used to cover babies who were positioned with their feet to the middle or sides of the crib. The safest arrangements were when babies were placed side by side at one end, or at opposite ends with their heads in the middle, allowing covers to be tucked in tightly under the end(s) of the mattress. Nowadays, with baby sleeping bags parents have less to worry about regarding loose covers. And co-bedding of twins helps parents to keep their twins with them at night, which reduces the risk of SIDS. This is an important consideration given that most twins are born prematurely and therefore are at increased risk.

Useful tip

Fewer people use blankets in their baby's crib now than they used to, but if you do, remember the "feet to foot" guidance, and tuck the sides of the blanket firmly under the crib mattress so that a baby cannot pull it loose. Be careful about using a folded blanket as this counts as multiple layers. If you use a baby sleeping bag, choose one with a tog-rating relevant to the temperature of the room, and be aware that adding extra blankets is not recommended.

Chest sleeping

Protecting babies' airways is important in other sleep contexts besides the flat, firm, level surface of a crib or Moses basket. One common scenario is when babies sleep on a parent's chest (which as we've seen, babies love to do). In this situation it is important the adult is awake and able to monitor the baby's breathing, ensuring their face is turned to one side and their chin is tilted upward so that their windpipe isn't compressed or kinked.[31] Being awake also means the adult can hold the baby in place, and prevent them from sliding, which sometimes happens when parents fall asleep with babies on their chests and wake to find their baby face down between the pillows or sofa cushions. Falling asleep with a baby on a sofa is particularly hazardous.

Intentionally taking risks

In some cases, parents choose to take risks despite knowing about them. When parents knowingly take risks with their baby's sleep environment, they are often making what seems to them to be a logical trade-off between sleep safety and disruption to their own sleep. In her PhD research, Dr. Lane Volpe found that adult and adolescent mothers made different trade-offs.[32] In a sleep-lab video study, she observed, for example, that several adolescent mothers used **bottle-propping** (holding a feeding bottle in place using pillows so a baby can "self-feed") while bed-sharing or room-sharing as a way to reduce the disruption to their own sleep. In contrast, several adult mothers who opted to place their babies in a separate bedroom used soft bedding, soft toys, and placed loose blankets near babies' faces to create a comfortable and comforting sleep space to help their babies sleep "well" and avoid the disruption of night-waking.[33] It is worth remembering that there are other ways to cope with baby-related sleep disruption that are safer for babies (see Chapter 9).

Making sense of risks

Despite all the research into risk factors, sleep safety and SUDI prevention, researchers still cannot explain to families exactly which babies are at risk, and precisely what they should avoid, although various models for SIDS have tried to do this.

In 1994 a group of researchers in Boston, Massachusetts, suggested an explanatory model for SIDS that drew together all the known risks associated with unexplained infant deaths.[34] The **Triple Risk Model** (Figure 7.1) emphasizes that for SIDS to

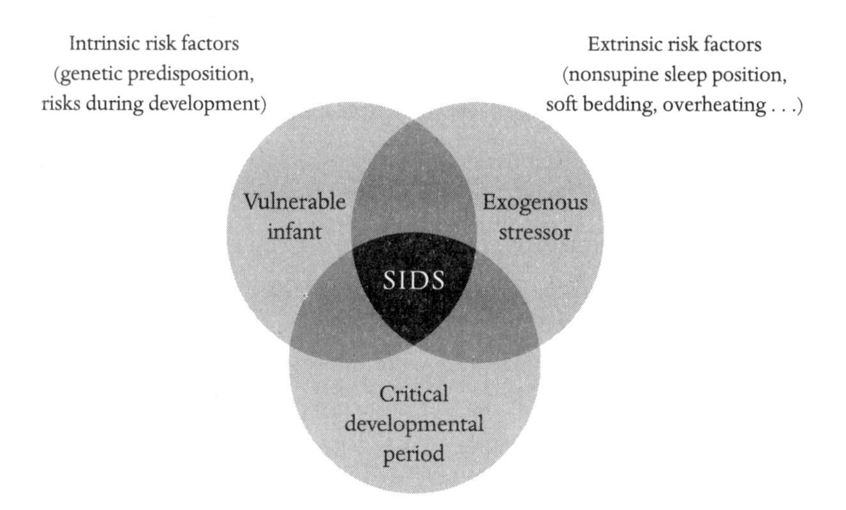

Figure 7.1 The Triple Risk Model for SIDS[35]

occur there is typically: a) a vulnerable baby, who b) is in a critical phase of development, and who c) experiences an external stressor that poses a physiological challenge that this baby is unable to overcome at this time. The vulnerability experienced by the baby may be prematurity, low birth weight, prenatal smoke exposure, or something that is only discovered after a baby's death, such as a brainstem anomaly or a genetic predisposition. The "critical developmental period" is between two and four months of age, which is when the majority of SIDS occur, and the external stressor can be any of the sleep risk factors, such as prone sleep position, lone sleep, overheating or airway covering.

According to the Triple Risk Model, SIDS happens if all three factors combine to create a situation from which a baby cannot recover during a particular sleep episode. A vulnerable baby who was outside the critical developmental period would not succumb, nor would a non-vulnerable baby, even if during the critical developmental period. This explains why some parents may have placed all their babies prone for every sleep with no ill effects—if these babies were not vulnerable, then their sleep position did not put them at risk. The difficulty we have is that not all vulnerabilities are readily apparent: a parent will know if their baby was born prematurely, of low birth weight, or had been smoke-exposed in pregnancy, and so can be extra vigilant about safe sleep to avoid external stressors, but if a baby has a hidden biological vulnerability such as a brainstem anomaly, a cardiac condition or a genetic predisposition, parents do not know that their baby's risk is increased. This is why SIDS reduction guidance is universally offered to all families; any of us might have a vulnerable baby, although this is very rare.

While the Triple Risk Model has been the main explanatory model for SIDS for the past 30 years, in 2024 another way of thinking about risks and protections was proposed by German pediatrician Herbert Renz-Polster and colleagues (including myself): the evolutionary-developmental model.[36] This offered an alternative explanation that considers an infant's vulnerability to SIDS as an imbalance between current physiological demands on, and current protective abilities of, a given infant. This perspective views SIDS as a developmental condition, occurring during the phase when neonatal reflexes have fallen away and self-protection abilities may not yet have fully developed. We argue that SIDS may be better understood if the focus on risk factors is complemented by a deeper appreciation of the protective resources that human infants acquire during normal development, when caregiving offers them the opportunities to do so, and propose that SIDS may reflect an evolutionary mismatch situation where some infants may encounter risks that they haven't had practice dealing with during their neonatal period when they are protected by reflexes. Rather than focusing only on the avoidance of risk, this model suggests how babies' resilience to risks may be enhanced by experiencing the protective skills associated with biologically typical behaviors such as breastfeeding and bed-sharing.

Co-sleeping and bed-sharing[37]

The Triple Risk Model helps explain why SUDI researchers have been concerned about co-sleeping, due to the potential for multiple "external stressors" to exist in this sleep environment (soft bedding, and head and airway covering). When co-sleeping was first identified in case-control studies as a risk factor for unexpected infant deaths, very little was known about how families co-slept or bed-shared, and how much variability existed. Guidance about SUDI and co-sleeping (which is defined as sharing any surface for sleep—safe or not) has been a source of anxiety and confusion for parents and health professionals for several decades, not least because the guidance varies from country to country, and even between organizations within the same country. While some differentiate between hazardous forms of co-sleeping (which include sofa-sharing and sleeping with a smoker or intoxicated adult) and safer forms of bed-sharing (such as breast-sleeping) in their studies, others lump all forms of sleep-sharing together as "co-sleeping," and recommend that all should be avoided, which obscures the fact that some forms are less hazardous than others, and denies parents the chance to make an informed choice about where their baby sleeps.

In some places, though, the guidance has changed in recent years as research has clarified specific hazards and benefits. In the UK, for example, the guidance around co-sleeping has been through several rigorous reviews and iterations since 2014, and there is now an emphasis on informed choice and individualized discussion with parents about their specific sleeping scenarios. In the U.S., on the other hand, avoiding all co-sleeping has been recommended through all iterations of SIDS risk-reduction guidance from 1997 to 2022.[38] These differences seen in national guidelines on co-sleeping can be explained, in part, by the specific evidence produced in each country that reflects who co-sleeps, and when, how and why they do it. It also relates to how SUDI rates are interpreted and understood by researchers and policy-makers in different places. In the U.S., and parts of Canada and Australia, for example, parents may be advised to never co-sleep or bed-share with any baby, or with a baby under three months of age, or with a smoke-exposed or premature/low birth weight baby. While the latter recommendation is universal given the intrinsic vulnerability of these babies, the others are contested for various reasons.

In the UK, the evidence from robust reviews of national case-control studies,[39] and from the National Child Mortality Database,[40] is that co-sleeping SUDIs occur in the presence of specific hazardous circumstances, involving sofas (very hazardous), parental use of drugs and/or alcohol (very hazardous), parental smoking, and premature or low birth weight babies.[41] Parents are therefore strongly advised to avoid any co-sleeping in these situations.[42] Outside of these known hazards, though, families are encouraged to make informed choices, with guidance taking a flexible and nuanced approach to helping parents figure out what works for them. The focus is on minimizing any bed-sharing safety risks rather than on avoiding bed-sharing altogether. Attempting to eliminate all risk by "banning" bed-sharing—an approach that was abandoned as a SUDI-prevention approach a decade ago in the UK—is unrealistic for most families. In our research studies parents have emphasized that attempting to follow dogmatic safe sleep guidance, especially when struggling with sleep deprivation, is impractical and too difficult. Sleep-deprived parents and babies may fall asleep together by accident, or in desperation, in hazardous situations such as on a sofa. Parents under the influence of alcohol or drugs may fall asleep with their baby unintentionally due to impaired decision-making, emphasizing that a sober adult should be in charge of the baby's safety at all times. In one of our studies we discovered multiple fathers coming home to sleep with their partner and baby on Friday or Saturday nights after consuming several pints of beer. In this situation, the safest solution would be for the dad to sleep elsewhere, but if under the influence of alcohol he forgets, then mom should remove the baby (and herself, if preferred) from the bed to another safe sleep space if they have one, or ensure she is positioned between the dad and baby if there is nowhere safe (i.e., not a sofa) that they can move to.

Nowadays in the UK it is recognized that most parents will sleep with their baby at some point. This might be intentional (planned or unplanned) or accidental, so encouraging parents to think ahead and make informed choices, while helping them to minimize any potential risks, is the safest option. This is known as **risk minimization**, in contrast to **risk elimination** (which as the name suggests attempts to eliminate all risks).[43] UK guidance, then, no longer advises to never share a bed with a baby but acknowledges that bed-sharing is a normal part of coping with nighttime infant care.

Due to the close link between breastfeeding and bed-sharing, it is unsurprising that a large proportion of parents who bed-share do so when their baby is under three months of age. However, some studies have found a possible increased risk for babies of bed-sharing during the first three months.[44] Babies are indeed more sturdy at the end of the fourth trimester than at the beginning; however, as we argue in our paper on the evolutionary and developmental perspectives on SIDS, in the newborn phase babies' risks from SIDS are reduced due to the existence of protective reflexes. Risks increase as newborn reflexes fade away in the second month, and learned protective behaviors (e.g., to defend airways) take over. Babies who bed-share from birth will have the opportunity to learn and practice these behaviors while reflexes still provide protection; however, babies who do not experience these opportunities (e.g., formula-fed solo sleepers) may be those most vulnerable to an unexpected external stressor (being placed prone or bed-sharing for the first time).

You may find yourself in a situation where bringing your baby into the bed is the only way you can calm them, the only way they will sleep, or you might find yourself with no other place for your baby to sleep. Bed-sharing might also be a culturally prescribed practice for you. Therefore, it is my belief that everyone with a baby needs to know what can make bed-sharing or co-sleeping hazardous, what to avoid and how to make it as safe as possible.

Useful tip

If you go out for the night, or host a party at home, plan ahead to ensure a sober adult is taking responsibility for your baby's safety for the entire night. This is because the effects of alcohol and drugs on adult sleep persist for a prolonged period (even until morning) and affect both your awareness and your judgment, potentially causing you to take risks with your baby's safety that you would never take when sober, as well as causing you to sleep more deeply with less awareness than usual.

Bed-sharing safety

If, and when, you bring your baby into bed, you need to know how to do so as safely as possible. While no one can guarantee a baby's safety (even in a crib designed for babies to sleep in), there are ways to enhance bed-sharing safety, such as placing babies on their back, flat on the mattress at breast or chest height, with the parent curled up around their baby, creating a barrier with their arm and legs, as shown in Chapter 6 (Figure 6.3). Bedcovers should be kept at the parent's waist so they cannot cover the baby's face or head, and you can wear a long-sleeved shirt or cardigan to keep warm. Babies should be dressed in the same clothing they would wear in a crib, with a sleeping bag or blanket (kept at baby's chest height or lower). Breastfeeding bed-sharing mothers tend to do these things automatically, but non-breastfeeding mothers, fathers and other family members may not. Keeping pets and other children out of the bed is advised as both may be less aware of the baby during sleep.

I am often asked about bed-sharing guidance for parents of twins—particularly for mothers who are breastfeeding. What is the safest way to sleep with two babies? This is not a question that can be definitively answered, as research studies have not looked at the SIDS outcomes resulting from different ways of bed-sharing with twins. As many twins are born prematurely and are therefore vulnerable, the safest answer is to tell parents of twins to never bed-share, and this is the position taken by most guidance. However, as we know with singletons, parents bed-share in order to cope with breastfeeding and nighttime care in a way that minimizes sleep disruption, and parents of twins experience this twofold. So for the purposes of minimizing risk while maintaining their sanity, what would the safer options for parents of twins look like? These suggestions come from parents themselves, who have taken part in our research and explained how *they* organized bed-sharing with twins, so you should consider these suggestions in light of your own circumstances and assess whether they would be suitable and safe for you and your babies.

The logically safest way to bed-share with twins is to do so one at a time—rotating both babies in and out of a bedside crib in turn; dads can play a useful role here as the rotator while mom lies and feeds her babies. Another option is for babies to be side by side in the bed, with mom curled up around the closer of the two, and rotating the babies from middle to outside so each can feed in turn. In this scenario it is important to make sure the outside baby can't fall from the other side of the bed. A bedside crib on the farthest side from mom, or a single bed for dad or grandma, is an option where families have sufficient space. I would avoid having one baby on either side of mom and rolling between them to feed as this means mom is always facing away from one of the pair; it is safest to be in a position where both babies can be observed simultaneously. Many mothers of twins learn to tandem feed their babies during the daytime (feeding both simultaneously), which is certainly less time-consuming than doing so sequentially, but with bed-sharing this causes difficulties as you need to sit upright, or be propped up on pillows with support under each arm to tandem feed two babies. This is not a safe position for sleeping, so if it is the only way mothers can feed and sleep during the early days of frequent feeding, it is crucial to have an alloparent monitoring the babies' safety, and moving them to a safe space, when mom inevitably falls asleep.

Useful tip

It is always a good idea to discuss co-sleeping safety (see Useful Tips below) along with other aspects of baby sleep safety with anyone who might care for your baby, day or night. Don't assume, for instance, that grandpa won't fall asleep on the sofa with baby on his chest in the afternoon while he is babysitting unless you discuss with him why it is important not to.

The crucial thing that anyone who might sleep with their baby should know is that risks vary according to *who* is bed-sharing or co-sleeping, *where* and *how* they are doing it, and *what* they have been doing before sleeping with their baby, as well as the intrinsic vulnerabilities that their baby may have been born with. The following example illustrates this.

In 2008–09 I worked in Bradford with pediatrician Dr. Eduardo Moya and the "Born in Bradford" study team to look at differences in SUDI-related baby-care practices among South Asian and white British families. Local data showed that white British families had a SIDS rate four times greater than the South Asian families—yet South Asian families commonly bed-shared, which at the time was strongly advised against. Eduardo and his colleagues wanted to gain a better understanding of what was driving this difference in SIDS. Our study participants were families that had enrolled in the "Born in Bradford" cohort study, which recruited 12,400 families during pregnancy;[45] 3,082 of these families completed our telephone survey (conducted in their preferred language) when their baby was between two and four months old. We found that the South Asian babies were much more likely than the white British babies to bed-share and to breastfeed, and much less likely to sleep in a room alone, sleep with a soft toy or sofa-share. These mothers never smoked, and no parents consumed alcohol. South Asian infant-care practices and lifestyles therefore protected babies from the biggest SIDS risks, and co-sleeping hazards such as smoking, alcohol consumption, sofa-sharing and solitary sleep, which explained the lower rate of SIDS in this community.[46] South Asian mothers were critical of UK sleep safety guidance at that time, and paid it little attention, pointing out that it was written "for the English mothers" and not the Asian mothers, as they could not recognize themselves or their cultural practices in the recommendations given.[47]

It is important, therefore, when considering SUDI risks that we think about the whole package of care a baby receives in all its cultural variants—who, from and how—as a dynamic set of interacting parts. Research studies, and consequently SUDI-prevention guidance, tends to fixate on isolated components of the larger picture, but parents are always balancing competing priorities and will mentally risk assess sleep safety as situations change and babies age.

Useful tips

When considering co-sleeping:

- Remember it is extremely hazardous to sleep with a baby on a sofa or armchair/recliner, after drinking alcohol, or after consuming (legal or illegal) drugs or medication that affects awareness during sleep.
- Be aware that bed-sharing with a parent who smokes (or a mother who smoked during pregnancy) increases the risk of SUDI, as does sleeping with a premature or low birth weight baby.
- Think about your bed and bedding with infant safety in mind (avoid gaps, soft surfaces, keep babies away from pillows, and do not swaddle or overwrap a bed-sharing baby).

- Make sure bed partners are aware the baby is in the bed, and do not allow small children or pets to sleep next to a baby.
- Make sure everyone who cares for your baby, day or night, is aware of this information.

Other sleep surfaces and products

There are a host of other things for parents to be aware of when baby sleep products and "nonstandard" sleep surfaces are brought into the mix. Car seats and bouncer seats, for instance, are not intended to be baby sleep spaces, but are often used as convenient containers for babies to sleep in. In particular, using car seats in the home is an issue.[48] When a baby car seat is in a car it tilts backward, and the baby who is in it leans backward, but when it is placed flat on the floor in the home it is more upright. In this position young babies can easily slump into a chin-to-chest position due to their poor muscle tone, which compromises the windpipe, kinking or compressing it, meaning babies are unable to get sufficient oxygen into their lungs leading to positional asphyxia.

Useful tip

Products that allow a baby's chin to drop onto their chest aren't safe for babies to sleep in; if they fall asleep in such a device, parents are encouraged to remove them as soon as possible and lie them on a safe flat surface.

Similar sorts of incidents with babies' airways can occur when using some slings and baby carriers—particularly bag-style slings that force babies' chins to their chests. When using a sling or baby carrier, always follow the manufacturer's instructions to ensure babies can't slump. Slings, wraps and carriers should be worn tightly to hold a baby upright against the adult's body, in a "chin off the chest" position with their back supported.

Useful tip

Baby-wearing consultants and volunteers at sling libraries are good sources of advice as to which kind of sling or carrier would be suitable for you and your baby, and can help ensure it is well fitted and you know how to use it safely.

There are other baby-care practices that parents often ask about regarding sudden infant deaths, but the data are not clear-cut enough to give guidance. One of these is the use of pacifiers, which are popular implements for calming babies, reducing crying and encouraging sleeping, although they can hinder breast-feeding initiation.[49] In some countries, such as the U.S., pacifiers are recommended for all babies as a SIDS reduction measure, but this is not the case in the UK, and there is no clarity around the mechanism by which the use of a pacifier might reduce SIDS.[50] Studies in the UK and Ireland have found that babies who are never given a pacifier do not have an increased risk, but that it is babies who normally have a pacifier and are without it on a particular night for whom the risk is increased. Therefore, in the UK, parents are advised that if they choose to give their baby a pacifier, they should use it consistently for every sleep for the first six months (avoiding the first month or so if initiating breastfeeding).

Swaddling is also used by parents to encourage their babies to be quiet and calm, and hopefully to sleep, and there are some concerns about whether swaddling is associated with SIDS or SUDI. At this time only four studies have looked at whether swaddling is a SIDS risk, two of which found it was, and two of which found it wasn't. This leaves us with no clear answer, but the level of risks associated with swaddling were found to vary according to the position in which babies were placed for sleep, being highest for prone and side positions.[51] There is also some evidence that swaddling is associated with shorter breastfeeding duration, and fewer arousals during sleep, both of which are linked to SIDS.[52] Contextual evidence therefore suggests caution in using swaddling, especially as a sleep promotion tool.

Baby sleep products are another common cause for concern. Many parents purchase or are gifted sleep nests or pods for their baby to sleep in, but reading the manufacturers' instructions often reveals they are only intended to be used when a baby is awake and being supervised and are not recommended for when a baby is sleeping. The problem with pods and nests is that the baby's sleep space is surrounded by a thick padded wall that: a) poses an overheating hazard by insulating the baby's head; or b) poses a breathing hazard if the baby's face is turned against the side. UK guidance suggests pods and nests are best avoided as there are no safety standards, other than for flammability, with which they are required to comply. In fact parents are often surprised to learn that there are no safety standards for most baby products on the UK market other than to ensure they are inflammable. The Lullaby Trust produces a useful leaflet about sleep products.[53]

Key things to remember about sleep safety

The information we have covered in this chapter on infant sleep safety can be scary and overwhelming the first time you meet it, but if you plan ahead with safety in mind, sudden unexpected infant deaths are very rare. I hope the information covered in this chapter will help you understand the risks and how to mitigate them. For most of us, practicing sleep safety becomes part of everyday baby care; knowing what to avoid and why is important in keeping your baby safe, even in unexpected circumstances, and you now know what you are aiming to achieve.

Very few of us will avoid exhaustion during early parenthood, and during these times we all struggle to stay clearheaded, so planning ahead for baby sleep safety is sensible. Sleep disruption is a predictable and normal part of learning to care for your baby. In the next chapter we will explore the different ways in which parents might try to cope with the sleep disruption that their new baby inevitably brings.

8. The darkest nights

Being a new parent is exhausting for many reasons, not least due to broken sleep, but before becoming parents many of us have little insight into how difficult this period can be. While the effect of a new baby on their parents' sleep is often the subject of jokes, memes and humorous comments, prolonged baby-related sleep disruption can have serious consequences for parental health, and consequently a baby's well-being. Whether it is framed as post-partum fatigue, baby-related sleep disruption, or the onset of postpartum depression, the experience of fatigue, tiredness and exhaustion touches almost all of us during the transition to parenthood. Why and how some of us struggle while others cope is something I became increasingly interested in over my career as I listened to the experiences of hundreds of new parents and explored the approaches for supporting people through this challenging period. While there is no doubt that all new parents experience some degree of sleep disruption during their babies' early lives, figuring out how to survive this period can be far from straightforward.

If you are reading this book in chapter order, you will know that young babies have very different sleep patterns from their parents, and that while sleep begins to consolidate at night after the first three months, when and how much this happens is hugely variable, meaning nighttime sleep disruption for parents often continues throughout the first year and beyond. Some baby-sleep authors and coaches advocate strict routines for babies during the first few months to "teach" self-settling and reduce sleep disruption for parents. Others advocate behavioral techniques to extinguish nighttime crying, and "train" the baby to stop signaling for attention during the night. Each "expert" will confidently tell you that their chosen method is the most effective, and indeed for many of these methods there is evidence (from individual anecdotes to rigorous trials) that they have worked for some families, but the criteria used to decide what "works" is very broad, inconsistent, and doesn't always mean what parents think it does. In this chapter we will explore what the various approaches entail, how they have been studied, and what "success" might look like. But before we get into that, we need to consider how postpartum fatigue and baby-related sleep disruption affect parents.

Parent–baby conflict is a fact of life

In contemporary Western cultures we are often led to believe the relationship between parents and babies—particularly mothers and their newborns—should be blissful, joyful and harmonious. Adverts and social media show us carefully curated images of maternal joy while relatives and strangers coo over our gorgeous baby, yet we might be feeling more stressed than blissful with a baby who seems to be more demanding than angelic. The first insight on this from evolutionary biology is that conflict between parents and their babies is predictable, and universal among mammals (and birds) who invest care in their young. It is normal to feel bored, overwhelmed and even resentful.

Parent–infant conflict can take many forms but basically means the following: it is in an offspring's own interests (in terms of their survival) to obtain as much **parental investment** for themselves as possible, by whatever means, for as long as possible.[1] In some species this might involve pushing their siblings out of the nest or displacing them from the mother's nipple. For human babies it may include nursing as often as possible, resisting separation whenever it occurs, crying persistently if separated from the caregiver, and prolonging breastfeeding duration (thereby suppressing ovulation and preventing the mother from conceiving the next child, who will take investment away from them).[2] While none of these behaviors happen consciously, and babies are not intentionally "manipulating" their parents, they have developed via the process of natural selection to ensure their survival needs are met; in other words, individuals who behave in these ways survive and pass on any genetic propensity for such behavior to subsequent generations.

In contrast, it is in a mother's evolutionary interest (given she has a finite number of reproductive opportunities) to modulate how much energy she invests in each child to ensure she can invest in other (current or future) children.[3] Mothers may use various (conscious or unconscious) strategies to reduce their input in response to their babies' requests for investment. For human mothers this might include initiating weaning, delegating carrying of babies to others, reducing the costs of nighttime care by bed-sharing, sharing the nighttime care of babies with fathers or others, and using pacifying techniques such as swaddling or pacifiers to suppress crying.[4] While men are capable of producing many more children than women, in most contemporary societies men father children with a limited number of partners and are likely to invest in those children.[5] Nighttime baby care can therefore become a key site of conflict not only between babies and their parents, but also between co-parents.

When we consider sleep disruption, an evolutionary lens can help us understand that babies' evolved biology prompts them to interrupt their parents' sleep and seek nighttime investment while parents' evolved biology influences them to minimize this disruption as much as they can.[6] Understanding this biological conflict can be helpful if you feel angry with your baby over sleep disruption,[7] or feel anxious that you and your baby should (but don't) have a consistently harmonious relationship. It will also help you remember why this normal parent–baby conflict sometimes spills over into conflict between parents,[8] which can cause further stress and anxiety.

What is normal adult sleep?

When considering the impact of our babies' sleep patterns on parents' sleep and fatigue, we need to think about what our expectations of our own sleep might be, and where they came from. Sleep habits in twenty-first-century Western societies are very different from those of our ancestors. The advent of electric lighting caused a huge shift in our daily activity patterns, allowing us to delay bedtime well beyond the onset of darkness, promoting what is known as **monophasic sleep**: sleeping in a single unbroken block. There is evidence from historical accounts of life in preindustrial societies and from contemporary human groups who live in non-electrified settings that, in the absence of electric light, sleep happens earlier in the evening, and is frequently **biphasic**: comprising two blocks of three to four hours each, with an extended period of quiet wakefulness in between.[9] This might, for instance, mean falling asleep around 8 p.m., sleeping until midnight, remaining awake talking, reading or thinking from midnight until 2 a.m., and then sleeping for another four-hour stretch until you wake for the day at 6 a.m. However, over the course of the past century or so, as we have illuminated the nighttime in industrialized societies, the opportunity for sleep has become reduced due to working patterns, increased ease of communication, and the availability of 24-hour entertainment, compromising biological rhythms and compressing sleep into a single monophasic period, which we now think of as normal.[10] In fact, we tend to associate "a good night's sleep" with unbroken monophasic sleep, and to consider a period of wakefulness in the night to be the sign of "a bad night's sleep." However, as we age and our sleep needs decline, many people find their sleep reverts to a biphasic (also known as a segmented) pattern.

As well as recent historical changes to sleeping habits, our current technologically dominated lifestyles make sleep an intensely monitored aspect of everyday life. The popularity of phone apps, watches and other "wearables" that keep track of our sleep means that new parents not only feel unprepared for the sleep disruption that a baby brings (as did prior generations), but the experience of sleep disruption and fragmentation is more closely recorded. We are now able to track and worry about aspects of our lives that prior to the advent of wearables, we only found out about if we had a sleep disorder and underwent a clinical sleep study. We are more acutely aware of our sleep patterns than we have ever been, and can compare our sleep last night with last week, last month and last year, in detail. Perversely, the huge emphasis now placed on achieving "good sleep" (according to the apps and monitoring devices' criteria for "good") can lead to anxiety and stress that promote insomnia. When personal sleep monitoring devices are used by new parents to track their own sleep or that of their baby, the chance of technological innovation fueling anxiety and obsession and promoting unnecessary stress is high.[11]

The impact of baby-related sleep disruption

The transition to parenthood is a time of extensive adjustment for families, made more difficult by altered sleep patterns. Many new parents report getting around half of the seven hours of sleep a night suggested for adults, with around a third being woken three times a night or more. For those who have spent their lifetimes to this point believing monophasic sleep is not only "normal" but also "required," the initial experience of disrupted, biphasic sleep is disconcerting.

During this period, parents in studies conducted by my team have described themselves as existing "in a zombielike state," "more tired than they've ever been in their lives before," with heightened emotions. Sleep-deprived parents suffer cognitive impairments such as concentration loss, and recount tales of driving to work in their slippers and falling asleep in the shower. Although superficially amusing, baby-related sleep disruption can be a serious concern, with a strong association found between baby-induced sleep disruption and parental depression, including increased severity of existing depressive symptoms.[12]

Sleep disruption contributes to the postpartum mental health issues that 15–20 percent of women who have recently given birth are treated for every year. And it is not just mothers who are affected. New fathers experience postpartum depression and anxiety disorders too, and have an increased risk of workplace and road-traffic accidents due to reduced vigilance and a greater propensity to fall asleep at the wheel. Babies are medicalized, medicated, and at risk from accidental and nonaccidental deaths, neglect and abuse when overwrought and exhausted parents choose any sleep over safe sleep, or perceive their baby as "naughty" or "manipulative" for waking at night and seeking parental attention, and—to extinguish night-waking—deny their baby a response. In extreme cases parents or other caregivers may lash out when they are unable to cope with middle of the night crying.[13]

Useful tip

While it is fine to take a break to calm down from the overwhelm of a crying baby, it is not fine to leave a baby without food or attention for prolonged periods. If you ever find yourself in a situation where you feel you may harm a baby out of frustration or desperation, put the baby in a safe place such as a crib or baby carriage, take a break, ask another adult to take care of the baby for a while, and seek support, especially if you feel overwhelmed or unable to cope.

One problem faced by Western parents is the entrenched cultural perception of normal infant sleep development, which has far-reaching consequences for parental and infant well-being. Inquiries as to whether a baby is a "good baby" who "sleeps through the night" are commonly posed to new parents, reinforcing a particular cultural view that prolonged baby sleep is important, should be achieved early, and that a night-waking baby is somehow aberrant. The need to have a "good baby" emerges as a way in which parents feel judged by society at large.[14] A failure to recognize that "normal babies" wake frequently during the night—and that they are doing so through need and not because they are misbehaving or manipulating their parents—makes such inquiries distressing for new parents, prompting them to question their parenting abilities, and whether they are damaging their baby's long-term health by failing to ensure they achieve sufficient sleep for optimal development.

In one of our focus group studies with UK families the issue of coping with sleep disruption came up spontaneously in response to questions about baby sleep. Participating parents declared how difficult they found it to experience baby-related sleep disruption for long periods, using dramatic terms like "nightmare" and "hellish." Mothers spoke of the ways in which lack of sleep interfered with their mental health, their physical health and their emotional stability.[15]

> I used to be very stressed-out because of that. I'd have him sleeping with me. Maybe on his own. Just feeding him something different at night [e.g., different formulas, cereals, etc.]. Anything.
>
> Sleep has been the biggest problem for me, like huge. First you get like delusional and things like that and you just... I ended up really, really poorly off, like... like I never slept an hour, more than an hour until she was about 6 months. I got myself really poorly.
>
> I was absolutely demented in the first 8 weeks.

While clinically diagnosed postpartum depression affects up to 20 percent of UK parents in the year following birth, there is evidence that up to 50 percent more experience mild to moderate symptoms.[16] For many of our study participants persistent sleep disruption negatively influenced their mood and day-to-day experiences of life, as illustrated by four young mothers in one of our focus group discussions.[17]

> Participant D: [When I don't get enough sleep] I just can't be trewed with nowt [bothered with anything].
>
> Participant B: It's horrible.
>
> Participant C: I've got no energy and...
>
> Participant D: Aye, you know that you've got all the bottles to do and dishes and if you think...

> Participant A: It makes you more depressed because you're just lying on the couch, and you can't be bothered and you're looking at all them bottles...

Our focus group participants found that their interactions with family members were also negatively affected by their experiences of sleep disruption and subsequent tiredness.[18]

> I get really crabby in the morning. It takes us a while... I mean, I'm a morning person but since I've had him, I'm tired. And it can, it can change how the whole day's going to be.
>
> I know if I've had a particularly bad night, I will be more short [tempered] with [my daughter] and shout, fly off the handle and then I feel terrible because it's not her fault it's just 'cause I'm tired.

Compared to the sleep they experienced during pregnancy, new mothers' postpartum sleep has been found to be more fragmented, shorter, less efficient (meaning more time is spent in bed to achieve the same amount of sleep), and associated with greater sleepiness and fatigue.[19] While researchers have only recently begun to examine the effects of these sleep disturbances, almost anyone who has parented a new baby will be familiar with the brain fog, sluggishness, irritability of frequent sleep disruption, and the annoyance, anger and anxiety that is provoked when others intimate that there might be something wrong with you, your baby or your parenting. In these moments—as difficult as it will be—try to remember that sleep disruption in early parenthood is unavoidable and temporary. You now have a good understanding of why it is normal; it is not a sign that you're a bad parent or you somehow have a "bad" baby, so don't allow anyone else's culturally laden perceptions make you feel otherwise.

Great expectations and cultural variations

Although babies all around the world have the same sleep biology, parental beliefs and practices relating to baby sleep vary widely. In the 2010 baby sleep industry-sponsored survey[20] of 30,000 respondents from 17 countries (discussed in Chapter 4),[21] the research team reported that in Asian countries babies and toddlers had later bedtimes, later rise times, less nighttime sleep and less total sleep than in Western countries. Bedtimes varied across countries by almost three hours, and sleep times by 100 minutes, although there were minimal differences in daytime sleep. In Western settings 57 percent of babies and toddlers were reported to fall asleep by themselves in comparison to just 4 percent of Asian babies and toddlers, and bed-sharing ranged in self-reported prevalence from 5.8 percent in New Zealand to 83.2 percent in Vietnam. Parental reports of sleep problems varied from 10 percent in Vietnam to 76 percent in China.

However, surveys can only obtain limited detail, and this one was particularly biased toward urban educated populations. Many smaller studies have examined cross-cultural differences in how parents perceive and respond to baby-related sleep disruption, documenting a wide variability in approaches. We have seen from Alma Gottlieb's ethnographic work that Beng mothers in Côte d'Ivoire were not particularly concerned about their babies' sleep.[22] Lying together at night, mothers did not keep track of how often their babies fed and, like bed-sharing mothers in our UK studies, were not entirely awake during night feeds. When babies woke their mothers at night, they were always offered the breast, and some babies clearly woke up more than others. According to Gottlieb, mothers described night-waking to be annoying at times, but also considered that it was normal, and responded to their babies without delay and in a matter-of-fact way.

Dr. Alyssa Crittenden, professor of anthropology at the University of Nevada, conducted interviews with Hadza hunter-gatherers in Tanzania, focusing on breastfeeding mothers who were habitually co-sleeping with their babies.[23] Although younger babies (up to six months) were said to feed "all night long," older babies (8–18 months) were reportedly fed once at night, and co-sleeping was not associated with sleep disturbance but was normal practice. As communal co-sleeping is typical for the Hadza, Crittenden and her team compared sleep quality for breastfeeding women, non-breastfeeding women, and men during communal co-sleeping, and found no differences between these groups, noting that sleep fragmentation was increased by having a greater number of co-sleepers (older children and men) together on the same surface. In subsistence societies where normal sleep arrangements are social, and sleep fragmentation is the norm, adapting to the nighttime needs of a new baby is less challenging as sleep is commonly fragmented by all sleep-mates. In Western societies, where we are habituated to sleep alone or in pairs, the disruption caused by a new baby comes as a shock because we are not used to experiencing sleep fragmentation.

Studies such as those by Gottlieb and Crittenden help de-center Western notions of baby care and reframe normalcy, illustrating that mothers and babies in nonindustrialized societies also experience baby-related sleep disturbances and do not perceive them to be problematic or in need of changing. This was also the case for some families in our focus groups, who described how having realistic expectations helped them overcome the challenges of sleep disruption: "Mothers should be aware before having the baby that, you know, there are going to be sleepless nights. And it'll be different"; while others physically adapted: "I think your body becomes used to sleep deprivation. I think it really does; I think you learn to cope on broken sleep. You learn to cope on five hours' sleep." Both perspectives imply that there are mental or attitudinal adjustments to be made that influence a parent's ability to negotiate this difficult period. One participant articulated this explicitly: "It's like from the beginning when I had my firstborn I thought he was a bit sleepless in the nighttime and then I just sat down and start realizing, if I won't accept this then I think this situation is gonna go worse for me, so I rather accept, and that, at the beginning of the situation, is how I managed to deal with my babies."

Of course, not all parents have the ability or insight to adjust their own mindset and reframe parent–baby sleep conflict as something to experience, accept and mentally minimize. Instead, many of us become fixated on attempting to find a solution and "taking charge" of our babies' sleep.

> I think you'll just do owt [anything], really, just to get them to sleep on a night 'cause...like, if they sleep, have a good night's sleep through the night, you're going have a good night's sleep through the night...rather than if you're up and down constantly all night, you're completely wore out the next day, you're going to be in a crappy mood and not want to do nowt [anything].
>
> I was asking me husband if we can do anything to, you know, make [the baby] a better sleeper [laughs]. Because your whole life depends on, you know, how they sleep, doesn't it? Only then can you do other work.

In Western countries where parents are expected to "take charge" of their babies and "teach" them how to conform to our cultural sleep habits and expectations, techniques for "fixing" a baby who disturbs their parents' sleep have not only flourished but become a huge business, particularly in countries where maternity leave is short or nonexistent for many women, and mothers feel under huge pressure to manage their babies' sleep from an early age in order to be able to return to work. There is a pervasive notion in many Western societies that it is the role of parents to "manage" their babies' sleep to ensure "good sleep habits" and optimal future development. It has deep historical roots and is the cause of much parental anxiety and guilt when we feel we are inadequate to the task. Remember, however, that the purpose of programs aimed at actively manipulating baby sleep is simply to make babies fit better into the adult worlds we have constructed.

Over 30 years ago when my first daughter was born I was working as a temporary lecturer at a large U.S. university where I was paid on a fixed-rate basis per course taught. There were no benefits attached to my post, including no maternity leave. I was allowed to take one week of "sick leave" while a colleague stepped in and taught my classes, and I was back in the classroom a week after giving birth. As previously mentioned, I had already made the decision to bed-share with my daughter, and I credit it, and the alloparental help of my sister-in-law, as being how I managed to survive as a working and breastfeeding mom during that year.

Useful tip

If you and your baby are coping fine or using other methods to harmonize your baby's needs with your own, baby sleep management techniques are not necessary, and it is OK to step back and allow your baby's biology to do its thing.

The narrative about "fixing" the baby's sleep to ensure "optimal future development" is another baby sleep myth. Whether sleep in early infancy is directly linked to later optimal developmental outcomes is impossible to assess; given all the many variables that one would have to somehow measure over the entire childhood of many individuals, such a study is unlikely to ever be undertaken.

"Fixing" the baby

As cultural contexts and expectations influence new parents' perceptions of baby-related sleep disruption, many parents seek the advice of friends, family or the internet (where a wild array of opinions will be proffered). Some seek the input of a clinician, hoping to be prescribed medication or a special diet to improve their baby's disruptive behavior, or turn to their health visitor, family nurse or (in the U.S.) their pediatrician for advice on **behavioral sleep interventions** they might implement. These interventions tend to be of two kinds: those that aim to prevent later sleep problems by teaching younger babies how to sleep "properly," and those that aim to resolve sleep problems in older babies so that they sleep "properly" too.

The most ubiquitous "solutions" to (arguably artificially created) baby sleep problems are products marketed directly to parents. These are advertised as magic wands that, once purchased, will surely make babies sleep blissfully for long periods; soft and comfy cushions and containers, rockers, swinging devices, hammocks, and even Wi-Fi-enabled electronic cribs are all advertised as promoting deep and peaceful sleep. More benign products such as baby bath liquid and massage lotion are marketed as sleep-promoting due to the inclusion of scents associated with relaxation, while warm baths and gentle massage help prepare a baby for the transition to sleep. Likewise, nighttime formula milks (which may only include added starch) are marketed to parents as products that will "help soothe and settle babies at the end of the day."[24] Corporate giants know babies are big business and new parents are an easy mark—especially if a product promises simple bedtimes and sleepful nights! But it is wise to be skeptical about any product or sleep practice that fosters deeper or longer sleep in babies six months and under, for reasons we have explored already.

Useful tip

In Chapter 7 we learned that practices and sleep environments that encourage deep and prolonged sleep in babies are linked to a greater chance of SIDS. Marketing for many baby sleep products tries to convince parents that prolonged and deep sleep is desirable for babies, often intimating that it promotes brain growth and thereby enhances cognitive development. Think carefully about these claims before buying or using these products, and remember that regular arousal from sleep provides protection from SIDS while Active sleep is when a baby's brain is growing and creating neural connections.

In some cases, parents might seek the services of a sleep consultant or sleep coach to help them resolve (perceived) baby-sleep issues. Sleep consultants and sleep coaches need no qualifications or accreditation to set up in business, so you need to be cautious about whose services you purchase, and ask about their training and background. They also offer many different approaches, so you need to be clear what sort of help you want and what fits with your personal parenting values. Depending on the philosophy of the sleep coach, their approach may involve education and adjusting parents' expectations, "tweaking" sleep arrangements, routines and behaviors until everyone is reasonably happy, or guiding parents through the implementation of a behavioral sleep intervention. In Australia, "Sleep Schools" offer parents weekend or weeklong residential courses in sleep training, and taking your baby to be sleep trained has become normative practice in some areas.[25] Other countries have highly paid sleep consultants who may even come to your home and sleep train your babies for you.[26] But in most instances parents who consider their baby has a sleep problem will turn to a self-help book or a parenting website or app, where they will find plenty of advice on how to "teach" or "train" young babies to sleep, and it is important to understand the difference between methods that "teach" babies to sleep and those that "train" them based on when and how they are implemented. The former are used in early infancy, prior to four months of age, and aim to encourage babies to learn how to self-settle so they can return to sleep without assistance when they wake at night. The latter are used after six months and use behavioral conditioning to extinguish signaling (crying) when babies wake at night. Parenting books and sleep consultants/coaches may offer "teaching" techniques, "training" techniques, or both.

Various methods have been devised for encouraging (or "teaching") young babies to fall asleep without parental help, and to return to sleep without parental input. Before we consider these methods, we might question the notion that babies need to be taught to fall asleep, or that sleep is a skill babies must learn. Babies are, after all, born knowing how to sleep—most of the time they are in the womb they are sleeping. What we are referring to here are methods used to "teach" babies to fall asleep in ways that are convenient for parents but incongruent with babies' needs or biology, such as to fall asleep without physical contact with a caregiver and to a parentally determined schedule. Both options emphasize parental control and management of baby sleep, heightening parent–baby conflict.

The methods used for "teaching" babies to fall asleep without parental help, and for settling themselves in the night, are often described as "preventative" behavioral interventions as they are intended to prevent rather than resolve perceived sleep problems. They aim to do this by increasing nighttime sleep during the first three to four months of life. Methods involve a delayed response when babies wake, and the gradual lengthening of intervals between feeds to provide opportunities for babies to return to sleep by themselves. In a widely cited UK randomized trial, these interventions were associated with a 10 percent increase in the number of babies who slept for five or more hours at night at 12 weeks,[27] an increase that was not considered sufficient for adoption as an intervention by UK health services.

Another commonly cited "technique" is to establish consistent and early bedtime routines. In a similar U.S. study parents were advised to avoid rocking or feeding to sleep, or using feeding as a soothing technique, to put babies in their own room by three months, reduce overnight feeds, and offer boring responses to night-waking (e.g., no speaking to the baby or eye contact). When compared with a control group of parents and babies who received a safe sleep intervention, the above techniques resulted in a 25-minute difference (on average) in parent reports of their babies' nighttime sleep duration at 16 weeks (four months). In later follow-up when babies were 40 weeks old (9–10 months), intervention group parents reported their babies slept, on average, 22 minutes more than those of the control group parents.[28] No information was provided on whether it was the same babies who were sleeping longer at each time point in this study. While an extra 25 and 22 minutes was statistically significant in the trial, I can't imagine it making a meaningful difference for many babies or families, especially as the averages disguise a large amount of variation, and there were no differences in sleep duration by the time the babies were a year old. It is always worth contemplating whether the effort needed to implement an approach to promote early settling is worth the presumed reward of longer parental sleep, when the benefit may be minimal, variable, and not guaranteed to last.

While preventative methods are often considered "gentle" because they do not involve leaving babies to cry for long periods, they can be harmful when implemented rigidly, especially if combined with strict feeding schedules that can result in underfeeding and failure to thrive.[29] If you choose to follow a preventative sleep routine with your baby from an early age, it would be best to do so flexibly and with caution, remaining alert to your baby's cues and not ignoring them in favor of following a sleep routine from a book, app or website.

In contrast to these preventative methods that aim to gradually teach babies how to sleep more like adults, sleep "training," or psychological extinction methods, are treatments that are intended to solve babies' sleep "problems." Although the context in which they are used may vary from country to country, the underpinning principles of sleep training or behavioral sleep interventions are basically the same, in that they aim to suppress an unwanted/undesirable behavior. Interestingly, the behavior that will be suppressed as a result of sleep training is not night-waking (as parents often assume) but signaling (crying) during the night. The goal of sleep training then is not more sleep for the baby, but less sleep disruption for the parent(s). There are pros and cons of these approaches, and it is interesting to examine parents' experiences of using them, including why some love them while others find them inappropriate, and even traumatizing.

Sleep training: The pros, the cons and the conundrums

In July 2023 I was invited to contribute to a symposium at the World Association of Infant Mental Health (WAIMH) Conference in Dublin. The symposium was organized by Professor Sarah Blunden from Adelaide, Australia, who had amassed a panel of researchers to speak about "The conundrums of behavioral sleep interventions in infants: Parental voices and choices." There were four of us on the panel: Professor Blunden and three invited speakers: myself (Durham, UK), Levita de Souza (Melbourne, Australia) and Macall Gordon (Seattle, U.S.). We arrived early to check our slides and confirm arrangements, and then waited patiently to see if any conference attendees wanted to hear what we had to say. By the time the session started, the seats were full, and latecomers were standing—behavioral sleep conundrums were clearly a hot topic!

Macall Gordon opened the session, addressing how sleep training methods are marketed to parents in the U.S. Although I lived in America for the entirety of my twenties, married an American and had my first child in the U.S., it was not until Macall's talk that I fully grasped what American parents are led to believe about baby sleep by mainstream media. In her talk she summarized the methods presented in 10 best-selling U.S. infant sleep manuals and websites, all of which advocate sleep training in one form or another, primarily using extinction and modified extinction methods (Figure 8.1). Guidebooks and parenting manuals, she told us, persuaded parents to sleep train their babies by asserting that sleep problems are common, potentially dangerous, persist long-term, and that sleep training is crucial to prevent "negative outcomes." Underlying themes included that "good parents" help their babies to sleep well, that starting sleep training early is most effective, and that extinction methods produce the most rapid results. According to the authors of these manuals, sleep training was quick, easy, and had no negative side effects.

Terminology	**Definition**
Unmodified extinction: popularly known as cry-it-out, cold turkey, tough love	No response provided to infant signaling (crying) during the night once settled alone for sleep at specified bedtime.
Graduated extinction (aka modified extinction, controlled crying, planned ignoring, minimal check): popularly known as Ferberizing, timed check-ins, pop-ins, camping-out, gradual withdrawal/disappearing chair	Strict behavioral response to infant signaling (crying) during the night once settled for sleep, involving parental checks at increasing intervals with minimal interaction, or with parental presence but no interaction and gradual distancing.

Figure 8.1 Behavioral sleep intervention methods advocated in U.S. infant sleep manuals for parents (summarized by Gordon, 2023)

To assess the accuracy of the claims made about these common sleep training methods Macall undertook a detailed review of behavioral sleep intervention studies published in peer-reviewed journals. She specifically focused on studies cited in systematic reviews, meta-analyses, and the American Academy of Sleep Medicine (AASM) practice guidelines, amassing 19 studies on unmodified extinction, and 27 on graduated extinction.[30]

Despite claims in the parent guidebooks that extinction is most effective when implemented "early," Macall found that only 2/19 studies of unmodified extinction involved babies under six months old, with 17/19 primarily focusing on the one-to-five-year-old age group. Likewise, only 7/27 studies of graduated extinction methods involved any babies under six months old, with 6/7 being only a small proportion of samples involving children up to five years of age. There was very little evidence that any form of sleep training with young babies is effective, safe, or (as is claimed) prevents "bad sleep habits." The studies that included babies under six months of age found that practical outcomes were small or nonexistent, had no significant impact on sleep, and their effects wore off over a few weeks. Despite multiple claims to the contrary, Macall could find no research into whether starting sleep training before six months is more effective than starting it later.

Extinction methods are based on American psychologist B. F. Skinner's principles of behaviorism: that a previously reinforced behavioral response can be extinguished by ignoring the behavior in question.[31] In behavioral sleep modification methods, responding to a crying baby in the night is considered to reinforce nighttime signaling for the parent's attention, and is extinguished by ignoring crying during the night and refusing to provide the desired response.[32] Multiple researchers have argued that such methods are inappropriate for babies under six months because, as we have discussed, night-waking is normal during at least the first six months, especially when a baby is night-feeding. Also, babies born prematurely will need to feed frequently at night for more weeks or months than if they were born at term. In addition, parentally perceived sleep problems may actually be undiagnosed feeding difficulties that should be ruled out before sleep issues are assumed to be the cause of frequent night-waking.[33] Furthermore, because it does not prevent sleep disruption in the long-term, multiple researchers have argued that sleep training in the first six months is inappropriately harsh treatment that will have to be repeated multiple times. Finally, sleep training methods that involve leaving a young baby to sleep in a room by themselves contradict SUDI prevention guidance, while specialists in babies' brain development warn that repeatedly triggering a baby's stress response via extinction methods in early life affects their emotional development.[34]

When examining claims about the effectiveness of extinction methods, Macall found "effective" meant different things to researchers and parents. Successful outcomes in extinction trials do not involve babies sleeping through the night, and most studies didn't measure babies' sleep. The primary outcomes of these trials usually involve reductions in maternal scores on postpartum depression scales, parental reports of improvements to their own sleep, and parental reports of less frequent disturbance by their babies. Even when parents reported better sleep for themselves, the sleep of their babies didn't change.[35] So if you are worried that your older baby is not sleeping "enough" (e.g., because they are waking during the night) and that this might compromise their cognitive or physical development in some way, be clear that sleep training is not the answer, as it does not actually help babies to sleep more.

While over 80 percent of extinction method trials report some kind of "positive outcome," most evidence (in terms of number and quality of studies) exists for toddlers and older children, not for babies. Moreover, in extinction trials only some families need a successful outcome for a method to be considered effective. As we've seen, positive outcomes involve relatively small differences in real life, such as parents gaining 20 minutes more (self-reported) sleep. For most extinction studies Macall examined, "success" primarily involved parents' perception of the sleep problem, and their perceived self-efficacy in controlling their child's sleep—parents felt that they had more control of their baby's sleep, and this was enough for them to deem the intervention successful. When objective sleep measures were used, though, actual child sleep outcomes were unchanged. Macall argues that parents purchasing sleep training manuals or web-based programs for use with their babies are rarely aware of the limitations of these methods.[36]

It's also worth noting that outcomes reported in clinical trials are difficult to replicate in real life. For instance, in Canada, 411 parents were surveyed about use of self-managed graduated extinction programs,[37] and of those who had used this method, almost half achieved no reduction in infant night-waking (signaling)—considerably less than the results seen in clinical and research trials. Although most research trials find extinction methods to be effective, in practice parents are unable to ignore their baby's distress for the duration needed for the method to work, and parental resistance to these methods has been documented for over 30 years. The reasons for parental struggle with extinction interventions have been categorized into seven themes relating to parents' ability to endure their child's crying, practical considerations around the disturbance to others, fear of repercussions such as damaging attachment, misinformation about appropriate use and expected consequences, incongruence with personal beliefs, different cultural practices and lack of culturally sensitive interventions, and parent wellness such as experiencing anxiety, depression or stress.[38]

There is ample evidence of both the pros and cons of behavioral sleep modification techniques. Some parents who have used an extinction approach with their babies encountered no difficulties and enthusiastically recommend it to others,[39] while for other parents "the treatment can be worse than the problem."[40]

Yet usually in marketing books and websites, and even in reporting the results of sleep training studies, it is only the positive outcomes that are emphasized or attract headlines. As Macall Gordon comments: "Extinction is 'the most evidence-based' method merely because it's the most researched, not because it's better. In fact, head-to-head, nothing works better than anything else."

This point was underlined by our colleague and symposium organizer at the Dublin conference, Professor Sarah Blunden of Central Queensland University in Adelaide, Australia, who found that compared to extinction, a more responsive approach to nighttime care, where parents attended to their babies' needs promptly, was just as effective, and involved less stress for both mother and child.[41] Sarah and her team evaluated stress, maternal depressive symptoms and sleep in mother–baby dyads who were randomly assigned to two different nighttime parenting methods (one responsive, the other extinction) and a control group. It is often claimed that sleep training involves just a few stressful nights, after which parents will sleep well; however, this trial found that sleep duration was no different between the three groups, but babies in the responsive group woke less (according to parental report), and mothers reported significantly less stress and fewer symptoms of depression. When parents attempt to implement sleep training outside the context of a research trial, they do not have access to the support and coaching provided by a research team, nor are they as consistent as when they are following a research protocol, leading to greater inconsistency, more stress and less chance of successful outcomes. Sarah concluded that responsive methods produce comparable outcomes to extinction (controlled crying) in terms of sleep outcomes, but from a relational and maternal mental health perspective, responsive methods are less stressful.

Useful tip

Given the wide range of different experiences parents report with sleep training, and the multiple variations of sleep training programs available, if you are thinking of using one of these programs with your baby, it is worth taking your time to find one you think has a reasonable chance of working for you. If it works as advertised and you achieve the outcome you are seeking, that's great. But if it doesn't, and especially if you are finding it stressful to implement, then there is no requirement that you persist. Experimenting to discover what works for you and your baby, and jettisoning what doesn't, is not "failing" at parenting—it is being judicious and flexible. You know yourself and your baby best, and you can make your decisions on that basis.

Educational interventions

In recent years there has been growing interest in parent–baby sleep from researchers and practitioners outside psychology—from anthropologists, sociologists, primary care and mental health practitioners, and public health experts. This diversity of perspectives has led to the exploration of new approaches that emphasize education and support for parents, such as my initiative with my colleague Dr. Charlotte Russell, the Baby Sleep Info Source or Basis website launched in 2012, which made anthropological and evolutionary perspectives on normal infant sleep freely available to parents.[42]

The advent of sleep education websites and apps prompted

interest in exploring educational approaches as preventative tools that were less costly and more acceptable to families than "traditional" bedtime coaching or sleep training interventions.[43] In designing educational interventions, helping parents to understand their baby's sleep behavior and how sleep develops over the first year has been a common starting point; however, sleep researchers from different disciplines are not yet on the same page in terms of the content of educational information that might be helpful to parents. While websites such as Basis made a legitimate attempt to offer parents educational information that was new and different, in multiple educational interventions researchers have assumed that giving parents "traditional" information about creating a "positive sleep environment" for babies (which typically involves placing baby alone in a crib with delayed parental responding to "teach" self-settling) would result in babies sleeping for longer and disturbing their parents less. But this is a questionable assumption, and the success of these programs depended heavily on the content and utility of the educational information parents were given. To understand why, let's look at three large parent education studies conducted in Canada, New Zealand, and Brazil.

In the 2010s in Toronto, researchers devised a 20-page booklet of information to support mother–baby sleep, offering information on self-settling techniques to promote sleep consolidation, such as using swaddling to reduce arousals, avoiding feeding and rocking to sleep, limiting social interaction at night, turning down the sound on the baby monitor (which implies babies were expected to be sleeping in a separate room) and implementing a bedtime routine. This information was discussed by child health nurses with a randomly selected group of parents in the first month postpartum.[44] Sleep was measured at 6 and 12 weeks and compared with those who did not receive the information. No meaningful differences were found between the two groups, with intervention mothers getting only six minutes more sleep than the comparison group when their babies were 12 weeks old—unsurprising with such an early follow-up, when the babies were too young to show much sleep consolidation. There was also a high proportion of breastfed babies in the sample, for whom frequent nighttime feeding would be typical at 6 and 12 weeks of age.[45] Although this was a well-designed and executed study, it missed the mark by uncritically assuming that "more sleep" is an achievable goal in the first 12 weeks of a baby's life, and so the information provided to parents was not useful to or usable by them.

In New Zealand, another team devised a parent education program to prevent "infant sleep problems" that emphasized self-settling and safe sleeping. This included information on the importance of developing a routine, responding quickly to "tired signs," placing baby down for sleep while awake and not rocking, holding or feeding to sleep, acting calm during night-wakings, delaying responding for short periods and responding in a consistent manner. Parent-reported baby sleep problems, sleep duration and night-waking were measured at six months.[46] Despite sleep outcomes being measured three months later than in the Toronto study, the New Zealand intervention did not prevent parent-reported baby sleep problems, reduce night-waking or increase sleep duration; teaching parents to encourage "self-settling" did not alter babies' sleep by any meaningful amount.

Our third example, in Pelotas, Brazil, was the first sleep education study in a low-to-middle-income country where cultural attitudes and practices around baby sleep differ from those in more wealthy English-speaking countries.[47] According to the study's authors, children in Brazil have later wake and bed times by approximately two hours and have high levels of bed-sharing with the mother compared to children in high-income countries. This study aimed to find out whether parent education here would improve babies' nighttime sleep in the first two years of life. The information covered sleep characteristics in the first year of life (e.g., how sleep duration and day/night sleep change with age), environmental factors that promote falling asleep (e.g., sleeping in a room on their own with "dim light and mild temperature," being put down "drowsy-but-awake"), establishment of a bedtime routine, and encouraging self-settling for both sleep onset and night-waking. But—just as in Toronto and New Zealand—no differences were found between the sleep education and comparison groups at 6, 12 or 24 months.

These three examples show that educational interventions using "traditional" sleep information do not help parents to "improve" their babies' sleep duration any more effectively than leaving them to cry (for shorter or longer periods). Given that none of these parent education interventions improved babies' objectively measured sleep outcomes this shows me that, unless there is an underlying clinical issue affecting sleep, babies will take as much sleep as they need. If we are going to support parents during this period of sleep disruption, we need to rethink the kinds of education and information that are needed. Instead of trying to increase baby sleep duration—it's worth saying again: babies will take as much sleep as they need—we might try to help parents in other ways, such as aligning more of their baby's sleep with their own sleep, using strategies that help them cope quickly and easily with sleep disruptions, and maximizing their own sleep by falling asleep as quickly as possible themselves, both at the beginning of the night and following baby-related night-waking. In fact, strategies for "self-settling" may be more usefully taught for parents to use on themselves rather than their babies.

Key things to remember about reducing parent–baby conflict

Parent–baby sleep conflict is a normal part of early childcare, but it can have far-reaching and negative consequences for both parents and babies. The traditional approach to date has focused on trying to manage or "fix" the sleep of babies so that they sleep more and disturb their parents less. Babies who don't comply with the expectations of their parents are deemed to have "sleep problems" that require treatment, and both the research and the public-facing discourse is dominated by behavioral interventions like sleep training. But, as we have seen, these interventions have, at best, only small effects on increasing babies' total nighttime sleep, and improving maternal mood, depression, fatigue and sleep quality, and either no or small effects on reducing night-waking.[48] If they work, they only work a little bit.

While some parents' inclination is that baby sleep should be modified to meet their needs, others prefer to try to meet their babies' needs and find different ways of coping with the inevitable sleep disruption.[49] Adjusting to their baby's sleep patterns seems to come more easily for some parents than others, and no single sleep intervention is likely to overcome all the challenges that parents face. It would make sense that a range of options be offered to parents as standard practice, yet as we have seen, the literature is dominated by extinction interventions, making it difficult for health professionals to offer alternative options and facilitate informed choice. Just as all babies are different, what works for each family will be different. There is no single way to "fix" baby sleep, because in most cases it simply isn't broken!

Thankfully, over the last decade, as the baby sleep paradigm has begun to shift, some researchers and clinicians have begun using new perspectives and trying out new approaches, and as we will see in the final chapter parents are at last beginning to have more options to choose from than just trying to modify their babies' sleep or simply waiting it out.

9. The sun also rises

There was no particular "breakthrough moment" with my own babies' sleep. Knowing very little about baby sleep back then, once I had made the decision to bed-share, nighttime care for us was mostly organic and instinctive. I did not have any baby sleep books and, as the internet involved dial-up modems and lots of waiting, I didn't have ready access to the opinions of others as we do today. With my first baby, my (U.S.) midwife endorsed bed-sharing while my grandmother-in-law advised me against it, and other than that I can't recall any direct guidance from anyone about my babies' sleep. My husband and I made it up as we went along, experimenting with different things until we found something that worked for us, and abandoning it if it didn't. I discovered early on that both my daughters were calmed by sucking, so after they were confident breastfeeders I gave them each a pacifier for a few months, which helped them fall asleep. Both lost their pacifiers when we were out and about in the second half of their first year, and I didn't replace them. By then I had learned lots of other ways of calming my babies, so the pacifiers disappeared with little protest, having served their purpose.

I never tried to "teach" my babies to sleep, though both my husband and I helped them to do so when needed, and we never considered them to have a "sleep problem," although we certainly often wished for more sleep. Their sleep patterns unfolded organically, sleeping wherever they were, whenever we slept, and with us throughout infancy. I couldn't tell you when my babies first "slept through the night," or how long they napped during the day; they just slept when they needed to and woke when they didn't, and we rolled through those first 365 days and nights together, only introducing changes to this approach (such as earlier bedtimes and bedtime routines) once our daughters had weaned from the breast sometime during their second year. My own experiences of not obsessing about sleep (primarily because I didn't know to do so was a thing) is one of the reasons I have found other people's accounts of struggling with baby sleep to be both fascinating and important to understand.

In mid-2016 I completed a three-year stint as head of my department and was released from university middle-management back into the wilds of academia—with an entire year of sabbatical lined up in which to resume the research I had mostly put on hold since 2013. What I had been longing to do was to devise and test a completely new approach to how we might support parents who are struggling to cope with their baby's sleep. Rather than letting them believe their baby had a sleep problem, telling them what they were doing wrong, and assuming all babies would respond to the same methods—as was commonly the approach in the existing literature—I wanted to create a tool kit of strategies from which parents could choose whatever they found effective at that moment, and then select something else when their baby's sleep patterns inevitably changed. I anticipated this would involve information about how sleep works, why babies need to feed frequently, how to bed-share safely, adjusting to fragmented sleep, reframing unhelpful thoughts, and why seeking help is so important.

I was fortunate to be able to draw on some of my previous work. As mentioned in the last chapter, back in 2011 my colleague Dr. Charlotte Russell and I had created the Baby Sleep Info Source (or Basis, as it became known) website, where we had summarized research about baby sleep from an anthropological perspective, and emphasized babies' evolutionary biology. Ever since its launch in April 2012 we had been receiving emails from health practitioners thanking us for providing a sensible source of information that they could direct parents to when they had questions about their babies' sleep.[1] But a website created by academics, while helpful for those who were happy to read about academic research studies, wasn't enough. The families who most needed help and support from health visitors were unlikely to read our website in detail (or at all). They needed something far more practical and user-friendly, advice that could be discussed in person with a trained practitioner who could offer individual support and encouragement over time.[2]

In search of sleep sanity

Before reinventing the wheel, good research should begin with a thorough search of what's been done before, to make sure the question you are burning to answer hasn't already been solved, or the approach you hope to use hasn't been shown to be ineffective. And so it was that I began the 2016–17 academic year rummaging around in the parenting and sleep intervention literature, looking to see whether the sorts of material I wanted to create were already out there. Chief among my criteria for the ideal project was that it could be easily delivered in the UK by health visitors and community nursery nurses (i.e., community health practitioners who support health visitors in their work), as this group of staff are on the front line when it comes to supporting parents whose baby's sleep is causing them problems, yet they receive little to no information about baby sleep or how to support these families in their training. What I found is summarized below, but first we need to understand where the information that typically reaches parents seeking help with their babies' sleep comes from, and how it is generated.

Parent-support approaches fall into two broad groups: those produced by academics or clinicians based on previous research evidence and evaluated using peer-reviewed studies; and those devised by popular authors based primarily on personal experience, anecdote and a smattering of scientific research. Some authors in the latter group claim their methods are based on research, which may involve feedback from panels of parents; however, these panels are typically made up of self-selected volunteers, and their feedback is not collected anonymously, or rigorously, or in sufficient numbers to be characterized as scientifically valid research. While these self-help baby sleep interventions may be individually helpful, and can be worth experimenting with, they are difficult to replicate and evaluate objectively because they are quite personal to the author and their particular parenting philosophy. If you have found a self-help approach that works for you, go with it. Here, however, I intend to focus on interventions founded in the peer-reviewed literature.

There were a few interventions of the type I was seeking in sleep-related areas. One example aimed at reducing postpartum fatigue called Wide Awake Parenting (WAP) was designed and evaluated by Dr. Rebecca Giallo, associate professor of psychology at Deakin University, and her colleagues in Melbourne, Australia.[3] Postpartum fatigue is characterized by an extreme lack of energy in the post-birth period, which may involve sleep disruption, but is also related to an exhausting birth experience and difficulties breastfeeding. Rather than focusing on advice about how to change baby's sleep, WAP focuses on supporting the parents. It is a practitioner-led intervention that offers support to mothers suffering with postpartum fatigue in setting goals, planning for and implementing strategies, and problem-solving barriers to saving and rebuilding energy. There is substantial overlap between the experience of postpartum fatigue and baby-related sleep disruption, such as how it affects the mental health of both mothers and fathers, increases stress, reduces parenting satisfaction and prevents enjoyment of a new baby. In supporting parents to devise and implement strategies for saving and rebuilding energy, the approach used by WAP highlights an important difference from the interventions we discussed in Chapter 8 for addressing sleep disruption. Here, the approach involves helping parents to manage activities and expectations—in short, to help them cope. WAP was underpinned by research that highlighted the relationship between maternal fatigue and inadequate social support, poor diet, poor sleep quality, and ineffective coping styles, including self-blame and disengagement, and helped parents to tackle these issues. As a consequence, WAP was effective in promoting mothers' self-efficacy to prioritize, plan for, and engage in health and self-care behaviors to promote their own mental health and manage their fatigue.

This was the sort of program I was looking for in terms of providing parents with active support strategies, but it wasn't tailored to address the specific problems parents face with baby-related sleep disruption, which often don't emerge until several months postpartum. Although WAP was not quite what I was after, I was encouraged that others were thinking along these lines and identifying useful approaches.

Translating Possums

I first heard from Dr. Pam Douglas, founder of the Possums Clinic for Mothers & Babies (now the NDC [Neuroprotective Developmental Care] Institute) in Brisbane, Australia, well over a decade ago. She told me that my work on evolutionary and anthropological approaches to parent–baby sleep had informed her own thinking on how to help parents understand and cope with their babies' sleep needs. I was delighted to find another baby sleep researcher that was on my wavelength. While I was wrestling with academic departmental management, Dr. Douglas—Pam, as I now know her—was developing and manualizing her Possums Sleep Programme with University of Queensland colleague Dr. Koa Whittingham. By 2016 their work had crystallized into several academic papers,[4] and was being used in clinical practice at the Possums Clinic where Pam (a GP) specialized in the care of parents and "unsettled" babies with feeding and sleeping concerns.[5] After reading dozens of intervention studies that failed to deliver what I wanted to accomplish, I found Pam's approach to be in tune with the scientific understanding of parent–infant sleep biology and our own anthropological studies of parent–baby sleep and parental needs during early infancy, and involved a similar approach to helping parents devise coping strategies that I had admired in WAP. To me it looked very much like the paradigm-shifting baby-sleep intervention we needed in the UK, and I wanted to know more.

The beginning of 2017 saw me on a plane from Newcastle, UK, to Brisbane, Australia, to spend six weeks immersing myself in what went on at Pam's clinic, finding out everything I could about her work on parent–baby sleep, from sitting in on consultations and talking with staff to interviewing parents about their experiences. Rather than teaching them how to "manage" their baby's sleep, Pam's focus was on helping parents to understand the behaviors and sleep biology of babies. The Possums Sleep Program helped new parents adjust their attitudes toward baby sleep, gave them confidence, reduced their stress and anxiety, and transformed their parenting journey, and Pam's patients loved it.[6]

Over the next couple of years Pam and I worked with my postdoctoral research assistant Dr. Catherine Taylor, pediatrician Dr. Vicky Thomas from the Great North Children's Hospital, and a group of practitioners and parents from the northeast of England, to create, test and evaluate a simplified version of the Possums Sleep Program that could be used by UK practitioners in their brief consultations with parents who had questions about their babies' sleep.[7] We called this new package *Sleep, Baby & You* (SBY), and it was based around a colorful visual discussion tool and engaging animations[8] that could be shared with parents during consultations to aid discussion and reinforce understanding. The animations were created especially for those parents who found reading challenging. In some settings (such as antenatal "preparing for parenthood" sessions), a midwife, health visitor or early help practitioner might use the *Sleep, Baby & You* antenatal discussion tool to encourage a group of parents-to-be to think about what baby sleep might look like, how it will change as their baby grows, and how they will deal with nighttime care. This might involve discussing how they will manage nighttime feeds, where their baby will sleep and what safe sleep will entail for their family, and who they can call on for help when needed.

When working with postpartum parents, practitioners use the *Sleep, Baby & You* materials to help a parent think through a particular issue they are struggling with, such as their baby waking early in the morning ready to start the day, and then develop strategies they might experiment with in order to alter or better cope with this situation, depending on their personal goals and preferences. This might involve delaying their baby's bedtime so they don't wake so early, reducing daytime sleep so they need to sleep for longer at night, bringing baby into bed for a feed to encourage another bout of sleep in the morning and meet their need to be with you, or the old favorite of blocking out the light (but this only helps if it is summer in a country where dawn happens early and baby is waking because of the light, and not some other reason).

In many cases practitioners use *Sleep, Baby & You* to reassure parents that their baby's sleep is normal and their coping strategies are sound, but where needed, talking through different ways of coping and finding enjoyment in the midst of postpartum challenges can make a huge difference. Most of the practitioner feedback we have received to date confirms that parents primarily want to know there is nothing wrong with their baby, and that they don't need to do something different just because someone has told them they should. Moms in our evaluation study commented:

> "Lovely nursery nurse Harriet[9] really helped me. One chat to her with the [SBY] leaflet took a huge weight off my shoulders, I've stopped trying to fix things that aren't broken, I just needed someone to tell me that my baby's routine is normal and to stop worrying all the time. Best leaflet I've ever read."
>
> "The nap info made sense and I'm still trying it, I didn't realize how little things could affect him."
>
> "[I have found] if I'm not stressed he seems to also be calmer."

Likewise, practitioners have found *Sleep, Baby & You* supports their work in encouraging responsive parenting, with one health visitor commenting: "I'm using it all the time, I think it's amazing, there's nothing that you teach that could do any harm, so why wouldn't you implement it? It's just so common sense, this is definitely the future."

After conducting an extensive evaluation with 164 practitioners who used *Sleep, Baby & You* in five UK locations,[10] and tweaking some elements in response to their comments, we began training

UK health practitioners, family workers, perinatal mental health teams and others to use the program in their work supporting families, and it is now being offered by a growing number of UK community health teams to support families in areas where parents have limited access to resources.

Certainly the Possums Sleep Program, and its offspring, *Sleep, Baby & You*, are not the only new-style parent–baby sleep approaches available, they are just the ones with which I am most familiar and can therefore talk most knowledgeably about. But it is very satisfying to see that a paradigm shift in baby sleep interventions, moving away from "fixing baby sleep problems" and toward acceptance of how babies sleep with appropriate parental support, is at last taking hold.

How can we put all this into practice?

Learning about how sleep works—about how our babies' biological needs, the evolutionary legacies of parent–baby conflict, the importance of contact and responsivity, the history of baby care—and the various ineffective approaches to "improving baby sleep" is all very interesting, I hear you say. But does it help me at 3 a.m. when my baby has had enough sleep for the night and is ready to wake the entire household? Does it help me juggle a toddler who wants to go to the park when it is baby's nap time? What about in the evening when I want to relax and my baby won't comply with their 7 p.m. bedtime? Are there any useful applications from the things you've talked about in this book?

Well, yes, there absolutely are!

The key thread running through this book is the importance of understanding that human evolution has resulted in baby humans whose brain development is exceedingly immature at birth. Human babies require prolonged and intensive care, and their needs are often in conflict with our own, which at times may seem to be more than we can handle. Yet simply knowing this can help us prepare for what's coming. The way in which our species adapted to meet this challenge evolutionarily and cross-culturally was via communal support for new parents and babies, through shared caregiving (or alloparenting).[11] We really aren't supposed to raise babies in isolation from our families or communities; seeking and accepting help from others is vital, and if we can set up support ahead of time, so much the better.

But accepting help—or even getting it in the first place—isn't easy, as I discovered when my first daughter was born in America, thousands of miles away from my family in the UK. New parents in twenty-first-century Western societies often find ourselves living and working far away from our closest relatives and friends, and finding and building new support networks can be challenging. In the meantime, the transition to parenthood is often unfolding in ways we did not anticipate. When we are seeking immediate solutions to the issues we are wrestling with it is easy to be seduced by products offering us "quick fixes" and the claims of social media "celebrities" promoting "easy" sleep training solutions. We need to have our wits about us at a time when we are typically feeling particularly witless. Hopefully after reading this book your wits are now on high alert.

What an evolutionary and anthropological view of parent–baby sleep tells me is that giving parents sleep information will not be effective if it simply repeats the same old messages about set bedtimes, putting babies to bed drowsy-but-awake, "teaching" babies self-settling, never bed-sharing, and avoiding feeding to sleep. The parents in our studies have found it useful to know that biological variation means all babies have different sleep needs that will change over time; this approach emphasizes that your baby is unique and so you should feel empowered to think outside the box, try new things, and figure out what helps you and your baby to reduce nighttime conflict and sleep as harmoniously as possible. Be reassured it does not matter whether you or your baby are doing the same as everyone else, so long as it works well enough for you, for now.

In the autumn of 2023 while I was writing this book, my research team was planning our annual contribution to the Festival of Social Science, an initiative funded by the UK's Economic & Social Research Council to help the public better understand what social science research entails and how it benefits society. We decided to host a parent-facing event with researchers and clinicians who focus on different aspects of baby sleep and who could address parents' questions from various perspectives. To begin, we used our social media networks to ask followers to submit questions about baby sleep (with a disclaimer that we wouldn't answer very specific questions pertaining to individual parents or babies due to lack of knowledge about their circumstances or specific health issues). From the 120 different questions received we created a long list of 30 topics that came up repeatedly; we then put these to a public vote to choose the top 10 questions for the panel to tackle.

Many of the topics raised spoke to parent–baby conflict, to the mismatch between cultural expectations and baby sleep reality, or both. Questions about transitioning away from contact naps, using products like swaddles and white noise machines, and having others be able to settle a baby all reflected the need of parents to somehow reduce their input into their baby's sleep at certain points over the first year—and all feed into parental wellbeing and mental health. While some babies have a temperament that will allow them to accept transitions in sleep arrangements easily, and will happily nap alone in a cot or crib after the most vulnerable period of the fourth trimester (the initial three months), other babies' survival instincts cause them to resist attempts to withdraw parental sleep support, even as their neurological competency increases between 6 and 12 months.

So, in this final section let's draw from all the different topics and issues discussed so far to help you think about how to put the concepts into practice via some of the most frequently asked questions by new parents. Here, we'll primarily lean on Pam Douglas's work,[12] along with my own, and highlight some of the key information we train practitioners to use in *Sleep, Baby & You*.[13]

Frequently asked questions

New parents are often puzzled about whether they should be actively doing something to help their baby fall asleep. There are many things we "could" do, but as Pam often comments, the role of parents isn't really to teach babies *how* to sleep (babies are born knowing how to sleep) but rather to remove the obstacles that stop them from sleeping. The buildup of sleep pressure triggers sleep onset, but it can only work when we are in a relaxed and receptive state, not when we are anxious, afraid or agitated. If we can help our babies (and ourselves) to achieve a calm and relaxed state, sleep will happen easily when sleep pressure is high.

How can I help my baby sleep?

For most adults, eating a good meal is an effective soporific, and this is also true for babies, who frequently nod off while being fed (assuming that feeding is a calm and relaxing activity for them; if there are feeding problems, then it may not be, and these need to be addressed first).[14] Although psychologists caution against allowing babies to fall asleep while feeding as this may cause an association between sleeping and feeding that means a baby will always need to be fed to sleep, this is unlikely if babies are encouraged to relax and drift into sleep in a variety of different ways. All around the world parents regularly use feeding, massaging, cuddling, stroking, walking, rocking and swaying to calm their babies so that sleep pressure can take hold; we could equally say that all around the world *babies* use contact with and movement by parents and other caregivers to help them relax and allow sleep pressure to tip them into sleep. If you experiment with what helps calm and relax your baby (often this is holding them, feeding them, making them feel safe and warm) and offer them opportunities to fall asleep in multiple ways and places, you will be making your life easier by not having to be tied to the same place, doing the same things, for every nap or bedtime (i.e., not "creating bad habits"!). And if your baby becomes familiar with multiple people calming and relaxing them in different ways from an early age, so much the better.

Does my baby need a regular bedtime?

During the first few months, when most babies sleep most of the time, a regular bedtime and pre-bedtime routine gives structure to the day, but mostly for the parents and other family members. Babies' developing circadian rhythm is influenced more by a regular wake time than a fixed bedtime, and there is no "ideal" time for babies to begin their nighttime sleep—only cultural conventions. "Ideal" is relative according to what parents are intending to achieve. If a baby's sleep pressure is not high when parents begin the bedtime process, then they could find themselves stroking, walking, rocking and swaying for ages before their baby is able to fall asleep. This is one of the pitfalls of insisting young babies have a fixed bedtime. What happens if a baby's biology is not ready for sleep at the time you've decided on (or have been told is when your baby "should" sleep)? You might spend a very long time implementing a "shush-and-pat" routine that gives you a sore back from leaning over the crib, when all you are really doing is passing time waiting for your baby's sleep pressure to rise. Or worse, you might spend days trying to create and implement the perfect nap schedule and optimize "wake windows" to ensure your baby is ready for bedtime "on schedule." I see this picture described repeatedly on social media by exhausted parents who have been persuaded that it is their job to "manage" their babies' sleep patterns but are finding the whole thing impossible due to the unpredictability of life; they are miserable and feel like failures.

A key component of Possums and *Sleep, Baby & You* is to empower parents to experiment with potential solutions and figure out which ones work for families, with an understanding that anything that works now may well need to be altered over time as babies mature and parents' needs change. Persisting with an approach that isn't working for you and your baby because it is "in vogue" or recommended by an influencer, expert or clinician is a recipe for misery. Seek out another option that you are all more comfortable with.

What if my baby just won't go to sleep?

In the scenario where babies are simply not ready for sleep at their allocated bedtime, try to forget the clock and interest them in something to engage their brain and senses to help promote the buildup of sleep pressure. If the weather is nice, a walk around the garden or down the street is an easy option, as there is so much more to engage a baby's senses outdoors than inside a static room with unchanging walls and ceilings. Pam talks about using "sensory nourishment" as a strategy for helping babies dial down—boredom from staring at the ceiling can be easily misinterpreted by parents as "tired cues," and sometimes babies need sensory input rather than sleep.[15]

On the other hand, if your baby's sleep pressure is high, and they are clearly ready to sleep but can't relax enough to achieve it (what in Western cultures might be called "overtired"),[16] then they need help to dial down and remove the block that is preventing sleep onset (fear, anxiety, pain, excitement, etc.). In this situation, contact, comfort and a calm, soothing environment may help some babies. Others respond to baby massage, to motion, or to being engaged in quiet conversation (they may not respond verbally, but babies most definitely respond to being talked to directly) and receiving your full attention. Try to stop and think about your own emotional and mental state when your baby is unsettled and can't unwind. Are they responding to your distress, frustration or distraction and trying to gain your attention and comfort? Could you put them in a sling or carrier and take them for a walk so you can both unwind a bit? Or ask someone else to do this while you do something relaxing for yourself or take yourself out of the picture for half an hour?

Can I stop my baby from waking just after I go to bed?

All babies will wake frequently at night in the early months, and this is something we should expect and prepare ourselves for. The impact can be reduced by keeping babies close at night, making night feeds as minimally disruptive as possible, and getting everyone back to sleep quickly and with minimal effort.

As they get older and their circadian rhythm starts to mature, babies might be very ready to comply with an early-evening bedtime, especially if they have consumed a large pre-bedtime feed. Their parents might put them upstairs in a quiet space (although as a reminder, before six months they shouldn't be left alone there) while they spend a few hours watching TV or catching up on the day. Babies' first sleep bout of the night is frequently the longest—perhaps four hours or so. Then the parents decide around 10:30 or 11 p.m. to go to bed. As we have seen, adults spend the first part of the night in deep sleep, with more REM sleep occurring during the second half of the night, so parents will likely be in the first part of their deep sleep phase when their baby wakes at the end of their initial sleep period (11 p.m. to 12 a.m. if bedtime was 7 p.m. or so).

Being awoken abruptly from deep sleep is disorienting and feels much worse than being awoken from lighter sleep and REM sleep. Aligning bedtimes to harmonize a baby's longest sleep period with their parents' first few hours of deep sleep could be a game-changer, accomplished by keeping the baby with you in the living room during the evening where the lights, the noise of the TV and conversation will keep baby napping rather than diving into their nighttime sleep. I might also suggest to parents to bring their own bedtime forwards by an hour or two if they don't want to keep their baby up too late. Remember to be patient—it might take babies a few days to adjust to this new pattern, but soon parents will be reaping the benefits of a decent bout of sleep before being woken, and sleep disruption in the second half of the night is much easier to cope with. Of course, this is just a temporary strategy until a baby's longest sleep bout lengthens and parents can slowly move their baby's bedtime earlier again if they want to—it might mean giving up your adult-only evening time for a few months, but it is a straightforward choice: better sleep or more TV time?

What do I do if my baby wakes at 3 a.m. ready for the day?

As babies move into the second half of their first year, they may appear to be done with sleep by early morning. Assuming we don't want to be getting up before the larks, there are a couple of ways to tackle this. We could decide to accept that this baby only needs so much nighttime sleep and delay their bedtime (as in the question above), so the entirety of their sleep time is shifted two or three hours later and they feel ready to start the day at a more sociable time. Or we could try to push some of their sleep period around the clock from daytime to nighttime (although this will not work until a baby has developed a day–night pattern) by reducing the length of daytime naps or eliminating naps altogether. We all have a certain amount of sleep we need in 24 hours, and some of us need more (or less) than others. If (for example) your nine-month-old baby only needs 14 hours' sleep in total, and they take two, two-hour naps during the daytime, they'll likely only need to sleep for 10 hours or so at night. Reducing those two-hour naps will mean more nighttime sleep and a later wake-up, which may be preferable for you. Alternatively, bringing baby into bed for a couple of hours early in the morning might encourage them to doze and snuggle for another hour or two, giving mom or dad the opportunity for a little extra snooze.

This issue also relates to the pitfalls of encouraging babies to take daytime naps in quiet, darkened rooms, and these becoming mini-nighttime sleeps that reduce a baby's sleep pressure back to zero (see below).

Does my baby need a consistent nap schedule?

Once your baby moves past the initial phase of sleeping around the clock and begins to start taking more of their sleep at night and having longer bouts of wakefulness during the day, you may wonder what you should be doing about naps. Popular advice often encourages parents to "teach" their baby to sleep in a crib by placing them in their crib for every sleep, daytime and nighttime. As a result, many parents, particularly mothers, become trapped by a daytime nap schedule that keeps them tied to the house. One of the key components of the Possums and *Sleep, Baby & You* approach to baby sleep is to forget about nap schedules and long daytime naps in cribs, and to instead let babies nap on the go, in the daylight, taking the edge off their sleep pressure as the day goes on but never dropping it all the way back to zero. Keeping sleep pressure rising until nighttime supports the consolidation of nighttime sleep and helps reduce night-waking.

Understanding that prolonged, dark, crib-based naps can, in fact, hinder nighttime sleep can be incredibly liberating, as having babies sleep on the go prevents their caregiver being confined to the home during nap times. Mental health is much improved when a caregiving parent can get out of the house daily to meet with friends, attend a group, walk the dog, or take an older child to a park or play area—in these scenarios the baby simply goes along and naps as and when needed, and when they wake they will have the rich sensory experience of being outdoors or in a vibrant environment to help keep their sleep pressure rising.

Pam encourages the mothers she works with to spend time on the weekend making a plan for what they will do to ensure they and their baby get out of the house every day during the subsequent week (walking around the shops, meeting a friend for coffee, attending a mom and baby group, visiting a market, dropping in on a relative, etc.). It is much easier to implement a previously made plan than it is to think of where to go or what to do in the moment, when doing nothing becomes the easier option.

How will I know whether night-waking is a problem?

It is normal, of course, for babies to wake for feeds every couple of hours day and night in the first few months, and one very practical way to cope with this is to bed-share at least part of the night if this can be done safely. Bed-sharing certainly saved my sanity and allowed me to breastfeed my daughters well into their second year, despite returning to work after a short period. But if a baby is waking in the night at hourly or shorter intervals, this may be a sign that all is not well—it may be an unrecognized feeding issue if it is happening in the first few months (in which case, see your local infant feeding health-care professional or a lactation consultant), but in older babies it may be a sign of disrupted circadian development, which can be a consequence of encouraging those long daytime naps in darkened rooms.[17]

Fortunately, this can be repaired by resetting a baby's circadian clock and supporting the development of their circadian rhythm. The former involves parents agreeing on a regular wake time for the baby and strictly implementing this (within a 10-minute window) for at least 14 consecutive days. This does not mean you should forcibly wake your baby at the same time every day, but you could expose them to daylight by opening the curtains and stimulate natural waking by starting to make the sounds of morning (turning on a radio, running a shower, etc.). After a few days a baby's body will begin to adjust to this activity and they will begin to wake at the new time.

It is important, however, to be consistent with this and not allow or encourage babies to wake later on weekends, for instance. The circadian rhythm can be supported by ensuring babies are exposed to daylight out of doors in the first half of every day. Going for a morning walk is an ideal way to do this. Light exposure in the morning prompts the suprachiasmatic nucleus (SCN) in the baby's developing brain to trigger the production of cortisol, which promotes alertness, and as daylight wanes, suppresses cortisol and promotes melatonin production that promotes drowsiness in preparation for rising sleep pressure to trigger sleep onset. Resetting and then supporting the circadian clock and avoiding darkness for daytime naps can help reduce night-waking.[18]

Why does my baby only want to contact nap? How am I ever going to get things done?

Meeting your baby's need for contact during naps does not have to mean finding yourself trapped under an increasingly heavy baby on the sofa for several hours every day. One solution is to meet a baby's survival need in another way. A baby's need for contact when napping might be accommodated by lying next to them on the bed or floor, allowing a parent to read, watch TV, text friends, answer emails, and so forth while they sleep. But if the problem is that you are feeling antsy about getting on with tasks, then wearing your baby in a wrap, sling or baby carrier (as appropriate for their age or weight) that allows you to move around and accomplish things can help resolve these feelings of being trapped. The carrying of older babies on their mother's back, or even giving them to another person to carry, is a worldwide practice that meets a baby's need for physical security and the mother's need to engage in household or economic labor, but it is one that has largely been lost from Western cultures. Sling libraries, baby-wearing groups, and many parent-support organizations can provide advice and help with choosing and fitting a carrier or sling and working out how to wrangle a baby into it.

Would swaddling my baby help them sleep?

Swaddling has been used by parents for centuries to simulate the feeling of being held, and some babies are pacified/settled by this form of motor restraint, which prevents them from flinging their arms or kicking violently and waking themselves from sleep during the first few weeks of life. Swaddling is one of those baby-care strategies that offers pros and cons: if overdone it can be hazardous, causing hip dysplasia (if babies are swaddled tightly with straight legs), reducing feed frequency (if babies' hands are restrained and they can't display feeding cues such as mouthing their hands), and increasing the risk of SIDS if swaddling continues past the first month of life (as swaddling suppresses arousal and promotes deep sleep).[19] Light swaddling around the shoulders, or the use of zip-up swaddling suits, which serve to prevent babies from flailing and startling but which aren't binding, can be helpful in the newborn period. However, it is important to remember to unswaddle a baby whenever they are fed or are taken into the parents' bed, as babies need their hands free to feed, and their arms and feet free to move covers, and sometimes parents, when in bed.[20]

How do I stop my baby from overheating in hot weather?

Most UK homes don't have air conditioning, and we don't normally experience temperatures above the low 20s°C (low 70s°F). However, in recent years the UK has experienced more frequent "heat waves," when the temperature in some parts of the country has reached more than 30°C (86°F). UK guidance states that the rooms in which a baby sleeps should be between 16 and 20°C (60 and 68°F). During these heat waves parents have wondered how to ensure their baby doesn't overheat. The Lullaby Trust advises parents to keep the curtains closed during the daytime to reduce the buildup of heat through the window, use a fan to circulate air (but don't point it directly at the baby), keep doors and windows open if safe to do so, and have baby wear only light, thin layers.

Babies lose heat through their heads, so it is important to ensure nothing covers a baby's head for sleep.

Will a red light help my baby sleep?

The key question here is "compared to what?" If your baby is happy sleeping in the dark, a red light will not improve this. But if your baby is older and afraid of the dark, a red night-light would be better than a white one, which emits wavelengths that can suppress melatonin and disrupt the circadian rhythm. Likewise, if you have a young baby who is waking frequently for feeds and diaper changes, trying to keep the room as dim as possible during nighttime activities is helpful in supporting circadian rhythm development, and so a red light might be useful here so you can see without exposing them (and you) to bright light in the middle of the night. However, if the question is about whether you need to purchase a red light product to "make your baby sleep more," or whether your baby needs one for their normal sleep development, then the answer is no. The current trend for selling red lights to parents of babies is just another marketing pitch. You may find one useful in specific situations as described above, but your baby doesn't *need* one. Like many products marketed to new parents, it is helpful to think about what it is you are being sold. If it is the promise of a baby who sleeps more and disturbs you less, be skeptical!

Are white noise machines helpful?

Like swaddles, white noise machines are commonly used to help babies settle more quickly into sleep and reduce night-waking. The machines mimic the sound of shushing (which some people liken to the whooshing noises of maternal blood-flow that babies are exposed to in the uterus). But remember that machines can shush much more loudly and for longer than a parent possibly can, and the noise they make never changes in strength or rhythm, so they can be overused in attempting to suppress a baby's normal arousal and feeding patterns. Placing white noise machines too close to a baby's head or having the volume too loud can permanently damage babies' developing hearing apparatus—so while they may be a useful tool for calming a baby occasionally, I would suggest they be used sparingly, and that human-produced shushing noises are preferable to mechanical or electronic ones. It may be helpful to bear in mind that using a tool or technique like this for every sleep, while seductive, can negate its usefulness for those occasions when babies may need a little extra help to fall asleep, and can quickly become a requirement for any sleep, meaning it is no longer a useful tool. If you are considering outsourcing the soothing and calming of your baby to a machine, weigh the pros and cons to both you and your baby of having a product do this or a human.

Is it OK for my baby to sleep in a sling?

Around the world millions of babies spend their days sleeping while strapped to their mother's body by a cloth or shawl of some kind, and although this has not been a common practice in Western countries in recent years, it is a very convenient one that is increasing in popularity. The use of slings and carriers (popularly known as baby-wearing) has not been the subject of much research to date, but some commonsense safety precautions have been recommended by baby-wearing aficionados in order to make sure slings are used safely.[21] The acronym T.I.C.K.S. is used to remind parents of the key principles of safe sling use, which involve ensuring the sling or carrier holds the baby:

Tight to the adult's body (to avoid them slumping down inside the carrier)

In view at all times (so the adult can see the baby and ensure their face is not covered)

Close enough to kiss (so the baby is positioned high on the adult's body)

Keep chin off chest (to avoid kinking and compromising baby's airway)

Supported back (so their tummy and chest are pressed firmly against the adult's chest)

When carrying your baby in a sling, be sure to consider the environmental temperature and the number of layers insulating your baby, as well as your own body heat, to ensure they don't get too hot.

Why will my newborn only sleep when I am holding her?

In our evolutionary past, babies who were happy to sleep alone would have quickly become victims of predation. Only sleeping when you are holding her is your baby's survival instinct as a primate mammal. No other species similar to us puts their baby down and leaves them in the newborn period; they are always in contact with their mothers, awake or asleep. Unless your baby is in contact with you, she cannot relax sufficiently to be able to sleep. Only on your body can she be sure she is safe.

Are wake windows important?

"Wake windows" do not form part of the science of baby sleep—this is a concept that has been invented by the parent-support community to (I think) simplify the concept of sleep pressure. The concept of wake windows assumes that at different ages babies are able to remain awake for a given period, after which their brains must sleep. Mothers are encouraged to time their baby's "wake windows" so they will know when their baby's next sleep period is approaching (with some added complications such as "wake windows" being shorter in the morning and longer in the afternoon). One problem with this concept is that it can disempower parents from recognizing how *their* baby shows signs of tiredness. Another is that it leads parents to think a baby's "wake windows" will be predictable and uniform when, in reality, sleep pressure builds up more or less quickly depending on brain activity levels. Sleep pressure is powered by adenosine levels (see Chapter 3), which are controlled by energy metabolism within cells—the more energy your brain uses, the more adenosine accumulates—so babies may build up sleep pressure more or less quickly depending on the intensity of their brain activity during periods of wakefulness, increasing the variation in duration of "wake windows" from one day to the next.

How do I know if my baby is waking because of digestive issues?

Feeding issues do sometimes masquerade as sleep issues, and these can be complex, requiring professional input to diagnose and resolve. It is important in early infancy to rule out feeding issues when a baby is waking frequently at night or having difficulty sleeping. However, many parents also assume that digestive issues such as reflux or colic are affecting their baby's sleep patterns when in reality their baby's sleep is typical and parents' expectations may be unrealistic. Behaviors that are interpreted as "colic" can reflect the need of babies to be helped to relax and unwind in order to be able to sleep, while many presentations of "reflux" can be resolved by offering babies smaller and more frequent feeds, and practicing responsive bottle-feeding in an upright position. Remember that tilting the baby's sleep surface has not been found to make any difference to reflux symptoms, and carries some risk due to babies' large and heavy heads being more likely to tip forward and kink their airways.

How important is "drowsy-but-awake"?

Trying to put babies in their crib "drowsy-but-awake" can be a futile activity. The idea is that a baby who becomes used to falling asleep in their crib will be more likely to return to sleep if they wake there during the night than a baby who falls asleep while feeding and then finds themself in the crib unexpectedly when they wake. While there is an element of logic in this suggestion the notion of drowsy-but-awake is not aligned with baby sleep biology. As sleep pressure increases, babies will be inclined to nod off as feeding (particularly breastfeeding) is soporific and their parents' arms are a safe and comforting place where they can relax. If you have a baby who is happy to reach drowsy but remain awake for long enough that you can put them in the crib, and you want to use this strategy, then please do so, but if your baby goes from drowsy to asleep before you can move from the chair, don't torture yourself trying to accomplish "drowsy-but-awake."

How do I know if my baby is going through a "regression" or a "leap"?

The notion of sleep regressions is discussed in detail in Chapter 4, where I suggest their origins in parenting literature arose in response to studies that showed some babies exhibit a period of consolidated sleep before resuming night-waking. This has been attributed to "developmental leaps," which may cause an increase in active sleep and arousal while a baby's brain is processing and encoding their new skill within their neural networks. However, none of these explanations are grounded in infant sleep science, and so-called regressions do not universally affect all babies or occur with predictable timing, so there are no evidence-based criteria for predicting or identifying "sleep regressions" or "leaps." In my view it is more helpful to recognize that baby sleep development does not unfold according to a strict timetable, and that night-waking and sleep duration progress more like a roller coaster over the baby's first year than a slow, gradual climb to the summit of a mountain.

What do I do if co-sleeping stops working for me?

As with all baby-care strategies, when something no longer works for you, switch tactics and try another way to harmonize your needs and those of your baby. You are the expert in what works for your family and should experiment with different options until you find the next thing that suits you all.

Why do false starts happen and how do I stop them?

"False starts" is a term used in the parenting literature to describe what happens when a baby wakes up 30–40 minutes after having fallen asleep, as if having had a short nap rather than having begun their nighttime sleep. There are several biological and behavioral explanations for this phenomenon. Biologically, it may be that your baby's sleep pressure was not high enough for them to transition into the next sleep cycle, and they have just taken the edge off their sleep pressure with a nap and are now ready to be awake again. In this situation, letting their sleep pressure keep rising for longer in the evening may be the answer, so experiment with keeping them awake for another half hour or hour before settling them for the night and see if this solves the problem. Or it may be that sleep pressure was moderately high, but they were not sufficiently relaxed and calm to be able to stay asleep at the end of their first sleep cycle. It might be worth trying techniques that you know calm and relax your baby at bedtime. But overreliance on the same tool or technique to help a baby fall asleep may only exacerbate the problem if a baby becomes accustomed to always falling asleep in a particular way.

Are short naps a problem?

In the newborn phase short sleep bouts during the day and night may signify an unidentified feeding issue and should be assessed by an infant feeding specialist. However, once babies are several months old and they are beginning to show signs of sleep consolidation (obtaining more sleep at night than during the daytime), then short naps are not a problem. As discussed above and in Chapter 3, short naps allow babies to take the edge off their sleep pressure while keeping sleep pressure building until nighttime. Although the saying "sleep breeds sleep" is often used to ensure babies get enough sleep during the day (naps) to prevent "overtiredness" at night, this is not supported by a biological understanding of sleep pressure.

Why do some babies only sleep for short periods for months on end while similar-age babies are snoozing for hours?

This reflects normal biological variation between individuals—some babies have greater sleep needs than others, and some exhibit more curiosity about the world around them. Babies have different temperaments and preferences from birth about many aspects of their lives, and sleep is no exception. Some will want to be held while others will be happy to be put down; some will be picky eaters while others will consume everything in sight; and some will prefer to sleep all day while others do not intend to miss a single trick.

How do I know if my baby is getting enough sleep?

Your baby is getting enough sleep if they are alert and happy when they are awake. While there is a lot of emphasis in popular science articles on the importance of sleep in infancy for learning and cognitive development, this is most relevant later in childhood when poor sleep patterns can affect memory consolidation and emotional regulation. During the first year of life, if your baby is alert and happy while they are awake, you do not need to worry about "optimizing" their sleep for future cognitive outcomes, so long as you are allowing them to take sleep when they need it and not restricting opportunities for sleep.

Obviously there is insufficient space here to explore how every sleep issue a parent may encounter with their baby might be reframed using evolutionary, biological or anthropological approaches, but hopefully you can see how these ways of thinking about baby sleep might add some useful perspectives for helping to understand how baby sleep works and offer strategies to parents who may need them.

Surviving the first 365 nights

The first 365 days and nights are some of the most crucial but exhausting for parents, not just because our uniquely vulnerable babies require care 24/7, but because immaturity at birth and rapid brain development mean sleep patterns change dramatically and often unpredictably as baby brains and bodies mature erratically in bursts rather than by a slow and gradual process. It might feel as though no two nights are the same—but despite what you may have been told or may have read, that is very normal.

Our understanding of how babies sleep during the first year of life has been shaped by the societies and cultures in which we live, the histories that have shaped those cultures, the changing needs of families over time, and the scientific paradigms that have influenced the study of, and recommendations about, baby sleep. We live in a world far removed from the circumstances in which our biology evolved and adapted, yet human babies are still helpless baby mammals, with a long post-birth developmental period, whose most fundamental need is the assurance that someone will take care of them until they are able to do so for themselves.

By exploring the evolutionary biology of parents and babies, exposing the origins of cultural assumptions and expectations of infant sleep, and examining how contemporary infant sleep practices are discouraged or reinforced, I hope this book has equipped you with the knowledge and information to make your own informed choices when presented with different options, opinions and conflicting recommendations.

Applying anthropological and evolutionary thinking to infant sleep and nighttime parenting does not produce a "quick fix" to make a baby sleep "better" or resolve new parent exhaustion, but it does help explain *why* we might feel exhausted and *want* a quick way to fix our baby's sleep. And when we are bombarded with "baby sleep solutions" from social media, advertisements, product manufacturers, and well-meaning friends and relatives, it helps if we stop and think about the nature of the "problem" they are offering us solutions for.

After decades of attempting to outsource infant care to technology, and to persuade new parents that their babies are the problem, the clear messages from evolutionary biology and anthropology are threefold: we need connection with other people to help with the challenges of nighttime baby care; we need to remind ourselves that normal baby sleep is hugely variable and that the intensity of babies' needs differs from one baby to another and over time; and finally, sleep practices around the world are hugely diverse and parents balance their own and their babies' sleep needs in a variety of different ways. How your baby sleeps over the course of their first year can happen in whatever ways work for you and your baby.

Glossary

Actigraphy: a method of monitoring sleep patterns using a device similar to a wristwatch that detects movement.

Active sleep: the infant equivalent of **Rapid Eye Movement (REM)** sleep, when a baby's brain is active. During active sleep, babies will often make noises, move around and open their eyes momentarily.

Alloparenting: cooperative caregiving encompassing any form of parental care by an individual who is not a direct parent of the infant being cared for.

Altricial: a bird or animal hatched or born helpless and in an undeveloped state.

Arcuccio: an Italian device from the 1600s resembling an arch over the baby that functioned as an in-bed co-sleeper to protect babies from their mothers' bodies during sleep.

Arousability: the ability to arouse easily (wake) from sleep, or shift from a deeper to a lighter sleep state, in response to an external stimulus.

Bed-sharing: the practice of sharing an adult bed with a baby or child. Compare with **co-sleeping**, which involves the sharing of any sleep surface.

Behavioral sleep interventions: commonly referred to as "sleep training," these generally involve extinction techniques designed to modify an infant's behavior during night-waking to eliminate signaling.

Behaviorism: a theory of learning based on the idea that behaviors are acquired or eliminated via conditioning by using positive or negative reinforcement.

Bicornuate uterus: a two-chambered uterus, found in multiple mammal species.

Biological sleep regulators: see **circadian rhythm** and **sleep pressure**.

Bipedalism: habitual walking on two legs. An evolutionary characteristic of hominins, including the evolutionary branch resulting in humans.

Biphasic sleep: a sleep pattern that involves two segments (also known as segmented sleep).

Bottle-propping: holding a feeding bottle in place using pillows so a baby can self-feed.

Breast-sleeping: the practice of mothers and babies sleeping together to facilitate nighttime breastfeeding.

Case-control method or study: a research method or study that compares two groups of people—those with the condition or outcome of interest (cases), and a matched group of people who do not have the condition or outcome (controls).

Circadian rhythm: the 24-hour "body clock" that regulates our cycles of alertness and sleepiness in response to changing environmental light levels.

Colostrum: the initial secretion from the mammary glands following birth. It is a thick yellowish fluid containing a high concentration of antibodies.

Co-sleeping: the sharing of any sleep surface with a baby or child. Compare with **bed-sharing**, which specifically involves the sharing of an adult bed. The broader definition of co-sleeping that includes room-sharing is not used in this book.

Cry-it-out: an extinction-based sleep training method that requires parents to put their baby to bed awake and ignore their baby's cries until they fall asleep.

Electroencephalography (EEG): a method for recording electrical activity in the brain by placing electrodes on the surface of the skull.

Encephalization: an evolutionary increase in the complexity or size of the brain or specific parts of the brain of a given species.

Ethnographic: studies typically conducted by anthropologists that involve prolonged familiarization with a society or cultural setting, primarily via participant observation.

Ethology/Ethologist: the science of studying animal behavior in natural settings by systematic observations. Ethologists are the scientists who conduct ethology.

Eutheria: the technical name for mammals who have a placenta attached to the uterine wall for supporting the in-utero development of the fetus.

Exterogestate: term used to recognize the characteristic of human babies to complete gestation outside the womb (exterogestation).

Extinction method: a psychological term describing the process of eliminating or reducing a learned behavior by withholding the reinforcing consequences that created or maintained it.

Feeding cues: pre-feeding behaviors expressed by newborn babies that serve as indicators of a readiness to feed, such as rooting, head turning, mouthing fingers and tongue clicking.

Fourth Trimester: the first three months of the postnatal period when babies and parents are adjusting to postnatal/postpartum life.

Hypnogram: a graph that represents the stages of sleep over a period of time.

Imprinting: innate learning in animals immediately after birth or hatching to recognize a primary caregiver.

Lactation: the production and release of milk by the mammary glands.

Marsupials: a type of mammal producing undeveloped young who are carried and suckled in a pouch on their mother's abdomen while they complete development. Found chiefly (but not exclusively) in Australia.

Monophasic sleep: sleeping for a single period in 24 hours. Compare with **biphasic** or segmented sleep.

Monotremes: a type of mammal that lactates but produces young by laying eggs. Monotremes do not have nipples and secrete milk from specialized pores.

Non-Rapid Eye Movement (Non-REM) sleep: also known as Quiet sleep, this is the phase of sleep when brain activity, heart rate and breathing slow down, body temperature drops, eye movements stop and muscles relax.

Parent–infant conflict: the evolutionary conflict arising over **parental investment** provided by a parent to an infant. Parents typically benefit from decreasing investment in any particular infant in order to invest in other offspring while infants benefit from increasing the parental investment they receive at the expense of any existing or future siblings.

Parental investment: in evolutionary biology, any parental expenditure (of time, energy, resources) that benefits offspring.

Placenta: a temporary organ produced in the uterus during pregnancy to convey nutrients and oxygen to the developing fetus and to remove carbon dioxide and waste products from the fetus to the mother's bloodstream.

Placental mammals: the common name for the **eutheria**—mammals who have placentas for supporting the internal gestation of the fetus.

Polysomnography: a study or test conducted during sleep to record physiologic aspects of sleep and wakefulness, including brain waves, breathing patterns and eye muscle movements.

Precocial: term describing the young of animal species born in a well-developed state of maturity and mobile shortly after birth or hatching.

Prone sleep position: sleeping on one's front, chest down.

Puerperal fever: a term coined in the eighteenth century to describe a postpartum infection, usually in the uterus, up to 10 days after giving birth.

Quiet sleep: the infant equivalent of non-REM sleep when babies are still, muscle tone is floppy and breathing is even.

Rapid Eye Movement (REM) sleep: a sleep phase characterized by increased brain activity, rapid eye movements, irregular breathing and rapid heart rate, during which dreaming typically happens.

Risk-elimination: an approach in SIDS/SUDI prevention that aims to reduce infant deaths by instructing parents to eliminate certain infant care practices such as bed-sharing and prone sleeping.

Risk-minimization: an approach in SIDS/SUDI prevention that aims to reduce infant deaths by informing parents about infant care practices that increase risk of infant deaths in particular contexts, and encouraging parents to make informed choices about the infant care practices they adopt given their particular context.

Rooming-in: the practice of keeping a baby in the same room as the mother or caregiver at night.

Rooting: an infant reflex (and involuntary feeding cue) where a baby searches for the nipple by turning their head, opening and closing their lips, and pushing out their tongue.

Self-settling: a baby's ability to move from an awake, alert state to sleep without any help from a caregiver. Sometimes erroneously called "self-soothing" (which is when children learn to regulate their own emotions, and which does not occur in infancy).

Simplex uterus: a single-chambered uterus, characteristic of some primates, including humans, that is accompanied by reduced litter size and increased body size of neonates.

Skin-to-skin contact: holding a newborn infant chest to chest on the mother's or father's bare torso immediately after birth.

Sleep architecture: the structural organization of normal sleep cycles that repeat over the course of the night.

Sleep consolidation: a process of sleep maturation in babies over the first year or so, involving the joining together of sleep cycles, compression of sleep into the nighttime, and reduction in night-waking.

Sleep pressure (or the sleep–wake homeostat): the accumulation of chemicals (adenosines) in the brain that trigger the feeling of sleepiness the longer we are awake.

Sleep problem: a parent-defined sleep difficulty in a baby, such as night-waking or inability to fall asleep at a predetermined time.

Sleep-related accidental deaths: infant deaths in sleeping situations, such as positional asphyxia, suffocation, entrapment or overlaying.

Sleep synchrony: a phenomenon where bed-sharing mothers and babies exhibit synchronized sleep cycles, which involve the shortening of the mother's sleep cycle to match that of her baby.

Sudden Infant Death Syndrome (SIDS): a baby death for which, after a full death scene investigation, consideration of a baby's medical history and a postmortem, no clear cause can be ascertained.

Sudden Unexpected Death in Infancy (SUDI): unanticipated deaths of babies that were healthy 24 hours previously.

Supine sleep position: sleeping on one's back, spine down.

Suprachiasmatic Nucleus (SCN): the "master clock" or pacemaker in the brain that regulates most circadian rhythms in the body.

Triple Risk Model: an explanation for SIDS-risk, encompassing three key factors: a vulnerable baby, a critical developmental period, and one or more external stressors.

Twilight Sleep: a combination of scopolamine and morphine administered to women in labor in the early twentieth century, which alleviated both the pain and memory of childbirth.

Ultradian rhythms: recurrent cycles repeated within a 24-hour period regulating biological processes such as hunger, thirst and heart rate.

Uspavani: a term used in the Czech Republic to denote the practice of parents calming and soothing a child (using various methods) to help them fall asleep.

Video-somnography: a video-based method to observe the sleep of one or more individuals and subsequently score sleep behaviors to obtain an objective assessment of sleep parameters.

Viviparity: the development of an embryo within the body of the mother and the birthing of live young.

WHO/Unicef Baby Friendly Initiative: an evidence-based approach to support breastfeeding and help parents develop close and loving relationships with their babies.

Zeitgebers: environmental cues that help regulate the circadian cycle and maintain synchrony between body and environment, such as daylight and darkness.

Acknowledgments

This book owes its existence to a large cast of colleagues, collaborators and friends who have willingly involved themselves in fostering an anthropological and evolutionary understanding of how babies sleep over the past 30 years, and to thousands of mothers, fathers and babies who graciously volunteered to take part in all manner of research studies during this time.

Special thanks go to Professor James McKenna, Professor Peter Fleming and Dr. Mike Wailoo, who have been the most generous and encouraging of mentors, and to the large cast of collaborators and coauthors I have had the pleasure of working with—you all know who you are. I am also fortunate to have supervised the work of a strong and dynamic group of postgraduate and postdoctoral researchers, each of whom made a distinctive contribution to the research I discuss in this book.

I am grateful to my editors at Cornerstone Press, Anna Argenio and Kate Craigie, and my agent at A. M. Heath, Tom Killingbeck, who inducted me into the world of popular science publishing with enthusiasm and kindness.

Most importantly, I am forever grateful to my husband and daughters, who not only provided my firsthand experience of how babies sleep but were also my guinea pigs, my traveling companions, my conference helpers, my bag carriers and my personal IT support. I am forever grateful to them for putting up with my baby sleep obsession and all its consequences.

Notes

Introduction

1 To quote Richard Smith, past editor of the *British Medical Journal*, https://blogs.bmj.com/bmj/2018/06/20/richard-smith-why-we-sleep-one-of-those-rare-books-that-changes-your-worldview-and-should-change-society-and-medicine/ who was paraphrasing Theodosius Dobzhansky in Dobzhansky T. (1964), "Biology, molecular and organismic," *American Zoologist*, 4: 443–52.

2 e.g., https://nina-kranke.com/back-to-the-stone-age-some-thoughts-on-evolutionary-explanations-in-infant-care/.

3 The Pleistocene is a geological epoch stretching from 2.58 million years ago to 11,700 years ago. The Paleolithic era, or "Stone Age," is an anthropological category pertaining to human prehistory covering roughly the same period.

4 https://www.nobelprize.org/prizes/medicine/1965/jacob/biographical/.

1. The helplessness of baby humans

1 Oftedal, O. T. (2011), "The evolution of milk secretion and its ancient origins," *Animal*, pp. 1–14. doi: 10.1017/S1751731111001935.

2 Langer, P. (2009), "Differences in the Composition of Colostrum and Milk in Eutherians Reflect Differences in Immunoglobulin Transfer," *Journal of Mammalogy*, 90(2), pp. 332–339. doi: 10.1644/08-MAMM-A-071.1.

3 "It naturally excites the idea of some deceptive preparation by artificial means," wrote English zoologist George Shaw in 1799. Shaw was the first to scientifically describe what turned out to be a very real creature.

4 Oftedal, O. T. (2011), "The evolution of milk secretion and its ancient origins," *Animal*, pp. 1–14. doi: 10.1017/S1751731111001935.

5 Martin, R. D. (2008), "Evolution of Placentation in Primates: Implications of Mammalian Phylogeny," *Evolutionary Biology*. Springer New York, 35(2), pp. 125–145. doi: 10.1007/s11692-008-9016-9.

6 Martin, R. D. (1992), "Primate Reproduction," in Jones, S., Martin, R. D., and Pilbeam, D. (eds), *The Cambridge Encyclopedia of Human Evolution*. Cambridge: Cambridge University Press, pp. 86–90.

7 Oftedal, O. T. (2000), "Use of maternal reserves as a lactation strategy in large mammals," *Proceedings of the Nutrition Society*, 59, pp. 99–106.

8 Lozoff, B. and Brittenham, G. (1979), "Infant care: Cache or carry," *The Journal of Pediatrics*, 95(3), 478–483. https://doi.org/10.1016/S0022-3476(79)80540-5.

9 Martin, R. D. (1992), "Primate Reproduction," in Jones, S., Martin, R. D., and Pilbeam, D. (eds), *The Cambridge Encyclopedia of Human Evolution*. Cambridge: Cambridge University Press, pp. 86–90.

10 Lozoff, B. and Brittenham, G. (1979), "Infant care: Cache or carry," *The Journal of Pediatrics*, 95(3), pp. 478–483. doi: 10.1016/S0022-3476(79)80540-5.

11 Small, M. F. (1998), *Our Babies Ourselves: How Biology and Culture Shape the Way We Parent*. New York: Doubleday Dell Publishing Group.

12 With acknowledgment that some birthing humans do not identify as mothers or female, "mother" is used here for consistency across species.

13 Martin, R. D. (1992), "Primate Reproduction," in Jones, S., Martin, R. D., and Pilbeam, D. (eds), *The Cambridge Encyclopedia of*

Human Evolution. Cambridge: Cambridge University Press, pp. 86–90.

14 Trevathan, W. R. and Rosenberg, K. (2016), *Costly and Cute: Helpless Infants and Human Evolution*. Albuquerque: University of New Mexico Press.

15 Rosenberg, K. R. (2021), "The Evolution of Human Infancy: Why It Helps to Be Helpless," *Annual Review of Anthropology*, 50, pp. 423–440. doi: 10.1146/annurev-anthro-111819-105454.

16 Gómez-Robles, A., Nicolaou, C., Smaers, J. B., and Sherwood, C. C. (2023), "The evolution of human altriciality and brain development in comparative context," *Nature Ecology and Evolution*. https://doi.org/10.1038/s41559-023-02253-z.

17 Dunsworth, H. M. et al. (2012), "Metabolic hypothesis for human altriciality," *Proceedings of the National Academy of Sciences,* 109(38), pp. 15212–15216. doi: 10.1073/pnas.1205282109.

18 Washburn, S. L. (1960), "Tools and human evolution," *Scientific American*, 203, 63–75.

19 Dunsworth, H. M. et al. (2012), "Metabolic hypothesis for human altriciality," *Proceedings of the National Academy of Sciences*, 109(38), pp. 15212–15216. doi: 10.1073/pnas.1205282109.

20 Trevathan, W. R. and Rosenberg, K. (2016), *Costly and Cute: Helpless Infants and Human Evolution*. Albuquerque: University of New Mexico Press.

21 Martin, R. D. (2007), "The Evolution of Human Reproduction: A Primatological Perspective," *Yearbook of Physical Anthropology*, 50, pp. 59–84. doi: 10.1002/ajpa.

22 Figure adapted from Martin, R. D. (1992), "Primate Reproduction," in Jones, S., Martin, R. D., and Pilbeam, D. (eds), *The Cambridge Encyclopedia of Human Evolution*. Cambridge: Cambridge University Press; and Martin, R. D. (1990), *Primate Origins and Evolution: A Phylogenetic Reconstruction*. Chapman Hall/Princeton University Press, London/New Jersey.

23 Ball, H. L. et al. (2006), "Randomised trial of infant sleep location on the postnatal ward," *Archives of Disease in Childhood*, 91(12), pp. 1005–1010. doi: 10.1136/adc.2006.099416.

24 Taylor, C. E., Tully, K. P., and Ball, H. L. (2015), "Night-time on a postnatal ward: experiences of mothers, infants, and staff," in Dykes, F. C. and Flacking, R. (eds), *Ethnographic Research in Maternal and Child Health*, pp. 117–140. Routledge.

25 Caudill, W. and Weinstein, H. (1969), "Maternal care and infant behavior in Japan and America," *Psychiatry*, 32(1), pp. 12–43.

26 Lee, K. (1992), "Pattern of Night-waking and Crying of Korean Infants from 3 Months to 2 Years old and Its Relation With Various Factors," *Developmental and Behavioral Pediatrics*, 13(5): 326–330.

27 Nelson, E. A. S. and Chan, P. H. (1996), "Child Care Practices and Cot Death in Hong Kong," *New Zealand Medical Journal*, 109: 144–146.

28 Tahhan, D. (2013), "Sensuous Connections in Sleep: Feelings of Security and Interdependency in Japanese Sleep Rituals," in Glaskin, K., Chenhall, R. (eds), *Sleep Around the World: Anthropological Perspectives*, pp. 61–78.

29 Barry, H. and Paxson, L. M. (1971), "Infancy and Early Childhood: Cross-Cultural Codes 2," *Ethnology*, 10: 466–508.

30 Whiting, J. W. M. (1981), "Environmental Constraints on Infant Care Practices," in Munroe R. H., Munroe, R. L., and Whiting, B. B. (eds), *Handbook of Cross-cultural Human Development*, pp. 155-179. Garland Press: New York.

31 Morelli, G. A. et al. (1992), "Cultural variation in infants' sleeping arrangements: Questions of independence," *Developmental Psychology*, 28(4), pp. 604–613. doi: 10.1037/0012-1649.28.4.604.

32 Wolf, A. et al. (1996), "Parental Theories in the Management of Young Children's Sleep in Japan, Italy, and the United States," in Harkness, S. and Super, C. (eds), *Parents' Cultural Belief Systems: Their Origins, Expressions, and Consequences*, pp. 364–384. London: Guilford Publications.

33 Cronin de Chavez, A. (2011), *Cultural beliefs and thermal care of infants: protecting South Asian and white British infants in Bradford from heat and cold*, Durham theses, Durham University. Available at Durham E-Theses Online: http://etheses.dur.ac.uk/3325/.

34 Cronin de Chavez, A., Ball, H. L., and Ward-Platt, M. (2016), "Bi-ethnic infant thermal care beliefs in Bradford, UK," *International Journal of Human Rights in Healthcare*, 9(2), pp. 120–134. doi: 10.1108/IJHRH-06-2015-0019.

35 Gottlieb, A. (2004), *The Afterlife Is Where We Come From*. University of Chicago Press. Available at: http://www.press.uchicago.edu/ucp/books/book/chicago/A/bo3620115.html.

36 Gottlieb, A. (2004), *The Afterlife Is Where We Come From*. University of Chicago Press. Available at: http://www.press.uchicago.edu/ucp/books/book/chicago/A/bo3620115.html.

37 Konner, M. (2016), "Hunter-Gatherer Infancy & Childhood in the Context of Human Evolution" in Mehan, C. L. and Crittenden, A. N. (eds), *Childhood: Origins, Evolution & Implications*. University of New Mexico Press, Albuquerque.

38 Hrdy, S. B. (2009), *Mothers and Others: The Evolutionary Origins of Mutual Understanding*. Belknap Press of Harvard University Press.

39 Sear, R. (2015), "Beyond the nuclear family: an evolutionary perspective on parenting," *Current Opinion in Psychology*, 7, 98–103. DOI: 10.1016/j.copsyc.2015.08.013.

40 Konner, M. (2016), "Hunter-Gatherer Infancy & Childhood in the Context of Human Evolution," in Mehan, C. L. and Crittenden, A. N. (eds), *Childhood: Origins, Evolution & Implications*. University of New Mexico Press, Albuquerque.

41 Hrdy, S. B. (2009), *Mothers and Others: The Evolutionary Origins of Mutual Understanding*. Belknap Press of Harvard University Press.

42 Sear, Rebecca (2021), "The male breadwinner nuclear family is not the 'traditional' human family, and promotion of this myth may have

adverse health consequences," *Philosophical Transactions of the Royal Society*, B 376 20200020. http://doi.org/10.1098/rstb.2020.0020.

43 Hrdy, S. B. (2009), *Mothers and Others: The Evolutionary Origins of Mutual Understanding*, p. 101. Belknap Press of Harvard University Press.

44 Hrdy, S. B. (2009), *Mothers and Others: The Evolutionary Origins of Mutual Understanding*, p. 109. Belknap Press of Harvard University Press.

2. *The curious history of babies in the nighttime*

1 Stearns, P. N., Rowland, P., and Giarnella, L. (1996), "Children's Sleep: Sketching Historical Change," *Journal of Social History*, 30(2), 345–366. http://www.jstor.org/stable/3789384.

2 Hardyment, C. (1983), *Dream Babies: Child Care from Locke to Spock*. Jonathan Cape.

3 Handley, S. (2016), *Sleep in Early Modern England*. Yale University Press.

4 Ekirch, A. R. (2001), "Sleep We Have Lost: Pre-Industrial Slumber in the British Isles," *The American Historical Review*, 106(2), 343–386. https://doi.org/10.2307/2651611.

5 An anglicized word used to describe a carrying vessel made and used by indigenous Australians.

6 A wooden or wicker carrying frame for babies used by indigenous North American and Scandinavian groups.

7 Stearns, P. (2004), *Anxious Parents: A History of Modern Childrearing in America*, p. ix. New York University Press.

8 Johnson, B. and Quinlan, M. (2019), *You're Doing it Wrong!: Mothering, Media, and Medical Expertise*, p. 4. Rutgers University Press.

9 Hardyment, C. (1983), *Dream Babies: Child Care from Locke to Spock*, p. 15. Jonathan Cape.

10 Boswell, J. (1998), *The Kindness of Strangers*. University of Chicago Press.

11 Hardyment, C. (1983), *Dream Babies: Child Care from Locke to Spock*, p. 24. Jonathan Cape.

12 Hardyment, C. (1983), *Dream Babies: Child Care from Locke to Spock*, p. 53. Jonathan Cape.

13 Walsh, J. H. (1857), quoted by Hardyment, C. (1983), *Dream Babies: Child Care from Locke to Spock*, p. 54. Jonathan Cape.

14 Boswell, J. (1998), *The Kindness of Strangers*. University of Chicago Press.

15 Unknown (1895), "The Arcuccio," *The British Medical Journal*, August, 380.

16 Handley, S. (2016), *Sleep in Early Modern England*. Yale University Press.

17 Hegele, A. (2018), "The curious history of sleeping through the night," *Synapsis*. https://medicalhealthhumanities.com/2018/07/10/the-curious-history-of-sleeping-through-the-night/.

18 Hardyment, C. (1983), *Dream Babies: from Locke to Spock*, p. 89. Jonathan Cape.

19 Tomori, Cecilia (2018), "Changing cultures of night time breastfeeding and sleep in the U.S.," in *Social Experiences of Breastfeeding: Building Bridges Between Research, Policy, and Practice*. Bristol: Policy Press, pp. 115–130.

20 Ball, H. L. (2008), "Evolutionary paediatrics: a case study in applying Darwinian medicine," in Elton S. and O'Higgins P. (eds), *Medicine and Evolution: Current Applications, Future Prospects*, pp. 125–150. Taylor & Francis.

21 Ball, H. L. (2008), 'Evolutionary paediatrics: a case study in applying Darwinian medicine', in Elton S. and O'Higgins P. (eds), *Medicine and Evolution: Current Applications, Future Prospects*, pp. 125–150. Taylor & Francis.

22 Apple, R. D. (1995), "Constructing Mothers: Scientific Motherhood in the Nineteenth and Twentieth Centuries," *Social History of Medicine*, 8(2), 161–178.

23 Hardyment, C. (1983), *Dream Babies: Child Care from Locke to Spock*, p. 125. Jonathan Cape.

24 Hardyment, C. (1983), *Dream Babies: Child Care from Locke to Spock*, p. 131. Jonathan Cape.

25 Hardyment, C. (1983), *Dream Babies: Child Care from Locke to Spock*, p. 132. Jonathan Cape.

26 Stearns, P. (2004), *Anxious Parents: A History of Modern Childrearing in America*, p. 46. New York University Press.

27 Ball, H. L. (2018), "The infant sleep myth," *Society Now*, 30: 18–19.

28 Hardyment, C. (1983), *Dream Babies: Child Care from Locke to Spock*, p. 173. Jonathan Cape.

29 Hardyment, C. (1983), *Dream Babies: Child Care from Locke to Spock*, p. 179. Jonathan Cape.

30 Hardyment, C. (1983), *Dream Babies: Child Care from Locke to Spock*, p. 185. Jonathan Cape.

31 Hardyment, C. (1983), *Dream Babies: Child Care from Locke to Spock*, p. 188. Jonathan Cape.

32 Hardyment, C. (1983), *Dream Babies: Child Care from Locke to Spock*, pp. 219–220. Jonathan Cape.

33 Gunderman, R. (2019), "Dr. Spock's timeless lessons in parenting," *The Conversation*, September 6, 2019. https://theconversation.com/dr-spocks-timeless-lessons-in-parenting-122377#.

34 Stearns, P. (2004), *Anxious Parents: A History of Modern Childrearing in America*, p. 167. New York University Press.

35 Blum, D. (2002), *Love at Goon Park: Harry Harlow and the Science of Affection*. Wiley.

36 Hardyment, C. (1983), *Dream Babies: Child Care from Locke to Spock*, p. 218. Jonathan Cape.

37 Winnicott, D. (1964), "Further thoughts on babies as persons," in *The Child, the Family, and the Outside World*, pp. 85–92. Harmondsworth, England: Penguin Books (originally published 1947).

38 Valentin, S. R. (2005), "Commentary: Sleep in German Infants—The 'Cult' of Independence," *Pediatrics*, 115(1), 269–271. https://doi.org/10.1542/peds.2004-0815J.

39 Hardyment, C. (2007), *Dream Babies:. Childcare Advice from John Locke to Gina Ford*. Frances Lincoln, London.

40 Hardyment, C. (2007), *Dream Babies: Childcare Advice from John Locke to Gina Ford.* Frances Lincoln, London.

41 Gettler, L. T. and McKenna, J. J. (2010), "Never Sleep with Baby? Or Keep Me Close But Keep Me Safe: Eliminating Inappropriate Safe Infant Sleep Rhetoric in the United States," *Current Pediatric Reviews*, 6(1), 71–77.

42 Barr, R. G., Bakeman, R., Konner, M., and Adamson, L. (1987), "Crying in !Kung infants: distress signals in a responsive context," *American Journal of Diseases in Children*, 141, 386.

43 Jolly, H. (1985), *Book of Child Care: Complete Guide for Today's Parents.* HarperCollins.

3. The sleep biology of babies

1 Widström, A., Brimdyr, K., Svensson, K., Cadwell, K., and Nissen, E. (2019), "Skin-to-skin contact the first hour after birth, underlying implications and clinical practice," *Acta Paediatrica*, 108(7), 1192–1204. https://doi.org/10.1111/apa.14754.

2 Foster, R. (2022), *Life Time: The New Science of the Body Clock, and How It Can Revolutionize Your Sleep and Health.* London: Penguin Life.

3 Walker, M. (2017), *Why We Sleep: The New Science of Sleep and Dreams.* London: Allen Lane.

4 Walker, M. (2017), *Why We Sleep: The New Science of Sleep and Dreams.* London: Allen Lane.

5 Bastani F., Rajai N., Farsi Z., and Als, H. (2017), "The Effects of Kangaroo Care on the Sleep and Wake States of Preterm Infants," *Journal of Nursing Research*, June;25(3):231-239. doi: 10.1097/JNR.0000000000000194.

6 Grigg-Damberger, M. M. (2016), 'The visual scoring of sleep in infants 0 to 2 months of age,' *Journal of Clinical Sleep Medicine*, 12(03), 429–445. https://www.ncbi.nlm.nih.gov/pmc/articles/PMC4773630/.

7 Rowan W. (1925), "Relation of light to bird migration and developmental changes," *Nature* (London), 115: 494–495.
8 Naylor E. (1985), "Tidally rhythmic behaviour of marine animals," *Symposia of the Society for Experimental Biology*, 39: 63–93.
9 Sanchez R. E. A., Kalume F., and de la Iglesia, H. O. (2022), "Sleep timing and the circadian clock in mammals: Past, present and the road ahead," *Seminars in Cell and Developmental Biology*, 126: 3–14. doi: 10.1016/j.semcdb.2021.05.034.
10 Joseph, D., Chong, N. W., Shanks, M. E., Rosato, E., Taub, N. A., Petersen, S. A., Symonds, M. E., Whitehouse, W. P., and Wailoo, M. (2015), "Getting rhythm: how do babies do it?" *Archives of Disease in Childhood*, Fetal and Neonatal Edition, 100(1), F50–F54. https://doi.org/10.1136/archdischild-2014-306104.
11 Iwata, S., Fujita, F., Kinoshita, M., et al. (2017), "Dependence of nighttime sleep duration in one-month-old infants on alterations in natural and artificial photoperiod," *Scientific Reports* 7, 44749. https://doi.org/10.1038/srep44749.
12 https://www.newscientist.com/question/how-long-can-you-go-without-sleep/.
13 http://handsonahardbodythemovie.com/.
14 https://www.imdb.com/title/tt0116481/trivia/.
15 https://theconversation.com/whats-really-going-on-when-a-child-is-overtired-and-how-to-help-them-go-to-sleep-194784.
16 Tinková, L. M. and Ball, H. L. (2022), "Lost in translation—the influence of language on infant sleep research," *Sleep Health*, 8(1), 96–100. https://doi.org/10.1016/j.sleh.2021.10.010.
17 Galland B. C., Taylor B. J., Elder D. E., and Herbison P. (2012), "Normal sleep patterns in infants and children: a systematic review of observational studies," *Sleep Medicine Reviews*, June, 16(3): 213–22. doi: 10.1016/j.smrv.2011.06.001.
18 Iwata, S., Fujita, F., Kinoshita, M., et al. (2017), "Dependence of nighttime sleep duration in one-month-old infants on alterations

in natural and artificial photoperiod," *Scientific Reports*, 7, 44749. https://doi.org/10.1038/srep44749.

19 St. James-Roberts, I., Roberts, M., Hovish, K., and Owen, C. (2015), "Video Evidence That London Infants Can Resettle Themselves Back to Sleep After Waking in the Night, as well as Sleep for Long Periods, by 3 Months of Age," *Journal of Developmental and Behavioral Pediatrics*, 36(5), 324–329.

20 Yoshida, M., Ikeda, A., and Adachi, H. (2024), "Contributions of the light environment and co-sleeping to sleep consolidation into nighttime in early infants: A pilot study," *Early Human Development*, 105923. https://doi.org/10.1016/j.earlhumdev.2023.105923.

21 Power, M. L. and Schulkin J. (2016), *Milk: The Biology of Lactation*. Johns Hopkins University Press.

22 Wright, P., Fawcett, J., and Crow, R. (1980), "The development of differences in the feeding behaviour of bottle and breast fed human infants from birth to two months," *Behavioural Processes*, 5(1), 1–20. https://doi.org/10.1016/0376-6357(80)90045-5.

23 Galbally, M., Lewis, A. J., McEgan, K., Scalzo, K., and Islam, F. A. (2013), "Breastfeeding and infant sleep patterns: an Australian population study," *Journal of Paediatrics and Child Health*, 49(2), E147–52. https://doi.org/10.1111/jpc.12089; Ball, H. L. (2003), "Breastfeeding, Bed-Sharing, and Infant Sleep," *Birth*, 30(3), 181–188. https://doi.org/10.1046/j.1523-536X.2003.00243.x; Rosen, L. A. (2008), "Infant Sleep and Feeding," *Journal of Obstetric, Gynecologic, & Neonatal Nursing*, 37(6), 706–714. https://doi.org/10.1111/j.1552-6909.2008.00299.x.

24 Gay, C. L., Lee, K. A., and Lee, S.-Y. (2004), "Sleep patterns and fatigue in new mothers and fathers," *Biological Research for Nursing*, 5(4), 311–318. https://doi.org/10.1177/1099800403262142; Montgomery-Downs, H. E., Clawges, H. M., and Santy, E. E. (2010), "Infant Feeding Methods and Maternal Sleep and Daytime Functioning," *Pediatrics*, 126(6), e1562–e1568. https://doi.org/10.1542/peds.2010-1269; Doan, T., Gardiner, A., Gay, C. L., and Lee, K. A. (2007), "Breast-feeding increases sleep

duration of new parents," *Journal of Perinatal & Neonatal Nursing*, 21(3), 200–206. https://doi.org/10.1097/01.JPN.0000285809.36398.1b.

25 Montagu, A. (1984), "The skin, touch, and human development," *Clinics in Dermatology*, 2(4), 17–26. https://doi.org/10.1016/0738-081X(84)90043-9.

26 Bowlby, J. (1969), *Attachment and Loss: Attachment* (Vol. 1). New York: Basic.

27 Blum, D. (2002), *Love at Goon Park: Harry Harlow and the Science of Affection*. Wiley.

4. Normal is as normal does

1 Ball, H. L. (2020), "The Mother-Infant Sleep Nexus: Night-Time Experiences in Early Infancy and Later Outcomes," in Gowland, R. and Halcrow S. (eds.), *The Mother-Infant Nexus in Anthropology: Small Beginnings, Significant Outcomes*, pp. 157–171. Springer. https://doi.org/10.1007/978-3-030-27393-4_9; Barry, E. S. (2021), "What Is 'Normal' Infant Sleep? Why We Still Do Not Know," *Psychological Reports*, 124(2), 651–692. https://doi.org/10.1177/0033294120909447.

2 Teng, A., Bartle, A., Sadeh, A., and Mindell, J. (2012), "Infant and toddler sleep in Australia and New Zealand," *Journal of Paediatrics and Child Health*, 48(3), 268–273. https://doi.org/10.1111/j.1440-1754.2011.02251.x; Sadeh, A., Mindell, J., and Rivera, L. (2011), "'My child has a sleep problem': A cross-cultural comparison of parental definitions," *Sleep Medicine*, 12(5), 478–482. https://doi.org/10.1016/j.sleep.2010.10.008.

3 Kohyama, J., Mindell, J. A., and Sadeh, A. (2011), "Sleep characteristics of young children in Japan: internet study and comparison with other Asian countries," *Pediatrics International*, 53(5), 649–655. https://doi.org/10.1111/j.1442-200X.2010.03318.x1.

4 Sun-Mi Chae, Ji-Young Yeo, Na-ry Chung, (2022), "A qualitative study of the sleep ecology of infants under 2 years old and their mothers in South Korea," *Sleep Health*, 8, 1, 101–106, doi.10.1016/j.sleh.2021.10.013.

5 Rudzik, A. E. F. and Ball, H. L. (2021), "Biologically normal sleep in the mother-infant dyad," *American Journal of Human Biology,* 33(5). https://doi.org/10.1002/ajhb.23589.

6 Rudzik, A. E., and Ball, H. L. (2016), 'Baby-Lag: Methods for assessing parental tiredness and fatigue', in L. L. Seivert and D. E. Brown (eds), *Biological Measures of Human Experience Across the Lifespan: Making Visible the Invisible* (29–46). Springer Verlag. https://doi.org/10.1007/978-3-319-44103-0_3.

7 Six months after writing this description I visited Beamish, a museum of northern life in County Durham, where a 1950s village had recently been recreated. Central to the village was the Welfare Hall, in one corner of which was displayed the paraphernalia of the baby clinics, and here, much to my joy and my daughter's bemusement, were the identical fabric screens on wheels, and noticeboards with developmental charts that I had recalled from my childhood 50 years ago.

8 The "Red Book" is the NHS-provided personal health record for each baby born in the UK, now increasingly becoming a digital record rather than a paper document.

9 E.g., Wonder weeks and Sprout baby.

10 https://www.babycenter.com/baby/sleep/how-much-sleep-do-babies-and-toddlers-need_7645.

11 https://www.happiestbaby.com/blogs/baby/first-year-sleep-schedule.

12 https://bibinoapp.com/en/blog/article/comprehensive-guide-baby-sleep.

13 Kleitman, N. and Engelmann, T. G. (1953), "Sleep Characteristics of Infants," *Journal of Applied Physiology*, 6(5), 269–282. https://doi

.org/10.1152/jappl.1953.6.5.269; Parmelee, A. H., Wenner, W. H., and Schulz, H. R. (1964), "Infant sleep patterns: From birth to 16 weeks of age," *The Journal of Pediatrics*, 65(4), 576–582. https://doi.org/10.1016/S0022-3476(64)80291-2.

14 Wolf-Meyer, M. (2012), *The Slumbering Masses: Sleep, Medicine, and Modern American Life*. University of Minnesota Press.

15 Newson and Newson (1963), *Patterns of Infant Care in an Urban Community*. Penguin.

16 Moore, T. and Ucko, C. (1957), "Night-waking in early infancy," *Archives of Disease in Childhood*, 32, 333–342.

17 *Better Homes & Gardens Baby Book*, 1965; *Good Housekeeping Baby Book*, 1956.

18 Henderson, J. M. T. (2001), *The Development of Infant Sleep: Implications for the Prevention of Infant Sleep Disturbance*. http://dx.doi.org/10.26021/9568.

19 Henderson, J. M. T., Motoi, G., and Blampied, N. M. (2013), "Parental expectations of infant sleep," *Journal of Paediatrics and Child Health*, 49: 535–540. https://doi.org/10.1111/jpc.12278.

20 Henderson, J. M. T., France, K. G., Owens, J. L., and Blampied, N. M. (2010), "Sleeping Through the Night: The Consolidation of Self-regulated Sleep Across the First Year of Life," *Pediatrics*, 126(5), e1081–e1087. https://doi.org/10.1542/peds.2010-0976.

21 The recommended age for introducing solids is six months. World Health Organization (2023) *WHO Guideline for complementary feeding of infants and young children 6–23 months of age*. https://www.who.int/publications/i/item/9789240081864.

22 American Academy of Pediatrics' *Guide to Your Child's Sleep* (1999), p. 1.

23 Crane, D. and Ball, H. L. (2016), "A qualitative study in parental perceptions and understanding of SIDS-reduction guidance in a UK bi-cultural urban community," *BMC Pediatrics*, 16(1), 23. https://doi.org/10.1186/s12887-016-0560-7.

24 Crane, D. and Ball, H. L. (2016), "A qualitative study in parental perceptions and understanding of SIDS-reduction guidance in a UK bi-cultural urban community," *BMC Pediatrics*, 16(1), 23. https://doi.org/10.1186/s12887-016-0560-7.

25 Crane, Denise (2014), *BradICS: Bradford Infant Care Study: A qualitative study of infant care practices and unexpected infant death in an urban multi-cultural UK population.* Doctoral thesis. Durham University. https://etheses.dur.ac.uk/10683/.

26 Ball, H. L. (2019), "Conducting Online Surveys," *Journal of Human Lactation*, 35(3), 413–417. https://doi.org/10.1177/0890334419 848734.

27 Mindell, J. A. et al. (2010), "Cross-cultural differences in infant and toddler sleep," *Sleep Medicine*, 11(3): 274 –280.

28 The article uses outdated racial terms "Asian" and "Caucasian" to characterize country-level populations, which I chose to not use and have instead used geographical descriptors with acknowledgment that neither are ideal; Shamambo, L. J. and Henry, T. L. (2022), "Rethinking the Use of 'Caucasian' in Clinical Language and Curricula: a Trainee's Call to Action," *Journal of General Internal Medicine*, May, 37(7): 1780–1782. doi: 10.1007/s11606-022-07431-6.

29 Mindell, J. A., Sadeh, A., Wiegand, B., How, T. H., and Goh, D. Y. T. (2010), "Cross-cultural differences in infant and toddler sleep," *Sleep Medicine*, 11(3), 274–280. https://doi.org/10.1016/j.sleep.2009.04.012.

30 Gottlieb, A. (2004), *The Afterlife Is Where We Come From.* University of Chicago Press.

31 Tahhan, D. (2013), "Sensuous Connections in Sleep: Feelings of Security and Interdependency in Japanese Sleep Rituals," in Glaskin, K. and Chenhall, R. (eds), *Sleep Around the World: Anthropological Perspectives*, pp. 61–78. Palgrave Macmillan.

32 Morelli, G. A., Rogoff, B., Oppenheim, D., and Goldsmith, D. (1992), "Cultural variation in infants' sleeping arrangements: Questions of independence," *Developmental Psychology*, 28(4), 604–613. https://doi.org/10.1037/0012-1649.28.4.604.

33 Wolf, A., Lozoff, B., Latz, S., and Paludetto, R. (1996), "Parental Theories in the Management of Young Children's Sleep in Japan, Italy, and the United States," in Harkness, S. and Super, C. (eds.), *Parents' Cultural Belief Systems: Their Origins, Expressions, and Consequences*, pp. 364–384. Guilford Publications.

34 Crawford, C. J. (1994), "Parenting practices in the Basque country: implications of infant and childhood sleeping location for personality development," *Ethos*, 22(1), 42–82.

35 Abbott, S. (1992), "Holding on and pushing away: comparative perspectives on an Eastern Kentucky child rearing practice," *Ethos*, 20, 33–65.

36 Alexeyeff, K. (2013), "Sleeping Safe: Perceptions of Risk and Value in Western and Pacific Infant Co-sleeping," in Glaskin, K. and Chenhall, R. (eds.), *Sleep Around the World: Anthropological Perspectives*, pp. 113–132. Palgrave Macmillan.

37 Tomori, C. (2014), *Nighttime Breastfeeding: An American Cultural Dilemma*. Berghahn.

38 Van Lennep, M. et al. (2023), "Age-dependent normal values for the 'Infant Gastroesophageal Reflux Questionnaire Revised,'" *European Journal of Pediatrics*. doi: 10.1007/s00431-023-05281-w.

39 Knowles, R. (2024), *Carrying Matters*. https://www.carryingmatters.co.uk/sling-safety-how-to-use-a-sling-safely/.

5. Hungry is the night

1 Hartmann, P. E. and Cregan, M. D. (2001), "Lactogenesis and the effects of insulin-dependent diabetes mellitus and prematurity," *The Journal of Nutrition*, 131(11), 3016S. http://jn.nutrition.org/content/131/11/3016S.short.

2 Hrdy, S. B. (2001), *Mother Nature: A History of Mothers, Nature and Natural Selection*, p. 129. Pantheon; Hayssen, V. (1993), "Empirical

and Theoretical Constraints on the Evolution of Lactation," *Journal of Dairy Science*, 76, 3213–3233.

3 Human Milk Foundation website: *Human Milk Science*. https://humanmilkfoundation.org/research/human-milk-science/.

4 Xu, R. J. (1996), "Development of the new-born GI tract and its relation to colostrum/milk intake: a review," *Reproduction, Fertility and Development*, 8(1), 35. https://doi.org/10.1071/RD9960035.

5 https://www.lllc.ca/newborns-have-small-stomachs.

6 Kendall-Tackett, K., Cong, Z., and Hale, T. W. (2015), "Birth Interventions Related to Lower Rates of Exclusive Breastfeeding and Increased Risk of Post-partum Depression in a Large Sample," *Clinical Lactation*, 6(3), 87–97. https://doi.org/10.1891/2158-0782.6.3.87.

7 Shel Banks, Infant Feeding Specialist, personal communication, October 2023.

8 Banks, S. (2022), *Why Formula Feeding Matters*. Pinter & Martin, London.

9 Sometimes a very forceful and prolonged milk-ejection reflex (MER) can produce a stream of milk into the baby's mouth that they struggle to cope with, causing them to arch away from the breast as they attempt to breathe and swallow. In this situation, taking the baby off the breast until the MER subsides, or feeding in a "laid back" nursing position can help.

10 Curiously, some baby sleep guidance advises against "allowing" babies to fall asleep during a feed so they can be put down "drowsy but awake." To a biologist this is a completely nonsensical notion, and one we will explore in Chapter 8.

11 Hardyment, C. (1983), *Dream Babies: Child Care from Locke to Spock*. Jonathan Cape.

12 Ball, H. L. (2003), "Breastfeeding, Bed-Sharing, and Infant Sleep," *Birth*, 30(3), 181–188. https://doi.org/10.1046/j.1523-536X.2003.00243.x.

13 Wright, P. M., McLeod, H., and Cooper, M. J. (1983), "Waking at night: The effect of early feeding experience," *Child: Care, Health*

and Development, 9; 9: 309–319; Zuckerman, B., Stevenson, J., and Bailey V. (1987), "Sleep problems in early childhood: Continuities, predictive factors, and behavioral correlates," *Pediatrics*, 80: 664–671.

14 Horne, R. S. C., Parslow, P. M., and Ferens D., et al. (2004), "Comparison of evoked arousability in breast- and formula-fed infants," *Archives of Disease in Childhood*, 89: 22–25.

15 Raphael D. (1976), "Night waking: A normal response?," *The Journal of Pediatrics*, 88: 169–170.

16 Rudzik, A. E. F. and Ball, H. L. (2016), "Exploring Maternal Perceptions of Infant Sleep and Feeding Method Among Mothers in the United Kingdom: A Qualitative Focus Group Study," *Maternal and Child Health Journal*, 20(1), 33–40. https://doi.org/10.1007/s10995-015-1798-7.

17 Rudzik, A. E. F. and Ball, H. L. (2016), "Exploring Maternal Perceptions of Infant Sleep and Feeding Method Among Mothers in the United Kingdom: A Qualitative Focus Group Study," *Maternal and Child Health Journal*, 20(1), 33–40. https://doi.org/10.1007/s10995-015-1798-7.

18 Centers for Disease Control and Prevention, *Breastfeeding Among U. S. Children Born 2000–2009*, CDC National Immunization Survey. http://www.cdc.gov/breastfeeding/data/nis_data/.

19 Bookhart, L. H., Anstey, E. H., Kramer, M. R., Perrine, C. G., Reis-Reilly, H., Ramakrishnan, U., and Young, M. F. (2022), "A nation-wide study on the common reasons for infant formula supplementation among healthy, term, breastfed infants in U.S. hospitals," *Maternal & Child Nutrition*, April, 18(2):e13294. doi: 10.1111/mcn.13294.

20 St. James-Roberts, I., Roberts, M., Hovish, K., and Owen, C. (2015), "Video Evidence That London Infants Can Resettle Themselves Back to Sleep After Waking in the Night, as well as Sleep for Long Periods, by 3 Months of Age," *Journal of Developmental and Behavioral Pediatrics: JDBP*, 36(5), 324–329. https://doi.org/10.1097/DBP.0000000000000166.

21 Manková, D., Švancarová, S., and Štenclová, E. (2023), "Does the feeding method affect the quality of infant and maternal sleep? A systematic review," *Infant Behavior and Development*, 73, 101868. https://doi.org/10.1016/j.infbeh.2023.101868.

22 Cohen Engler, A., Hadash, A., Shehadeh, N., and Pillar, G. (2012), "Breastfeeding may improve nocturnal sleep and reduce infantile colic: Potential role of breast milk melatonin," *European Journal of Pediatrics*, 171(4), 729–732. https://doi.org/10.1007/s00431-011-1659-3; Cubero, J., Valero, V., Sánchez, J., Rivero, M., Parvez, H., Rodríguez, A. B., and Barriga Ibars, C. (2005), "The circadian rhythm of tryptophan in breast milk affects the rhythms of 6-sulfatoxymelatonin and sleep in newborn," *Neuroendocrinology Letters*, 26(6), 657–661.

23 Doan, T., Gay, C. L., Kennedy, H. P., Newman, J., and Lee, K. A. (2014), "Nighttime breastfeeding behavior is associated with more nocturnal sleep among first-time mothers at one month postpartum," *Journal of Clinical Sleep Medicine*, 10(3): 313–319.

24 Doan, T., Gay, C. L., Kennedy, H. P., Newman, J., and Lee, K. A. (2014), "Nighttime breastfeeding behavior is associated with more nocturnal sleep among first-time mothers at one month postpartum," *Journal of Clinical Sleep Medicine*, 10(3): 313–319.

25 Montgomery-Downs, H. E., Clawges, H. M., and Santy, E. E. (2010), "Infant Feeding Methods and Maternal Sleep and Daytime Functioning," *Pediatrics*, 126; e1562; DOI: 10.1542/peds.2010-1269.

26 Rudzik, A. E. F. et al. (2018), "Discrepancies in maternal reports of infant sleep vs. actigraphy by mode of feeding," *Sleep Medicine*. https://doi.org/10.1016/j.sleep.2018.06.010.

27 Ball H. L. (2003), "Breastfeeding, bed-sharing, and infant sleep," *Birth: Issues in Perinatal Care*; 30: 181e8; Ball, H. L., Hooker, E., and Kelly, P. J. (1999), "Where will the baby sleep? Attitudes and practices of new and experienced parents regarding cosleeping with their newborn infants," *American Anthropologist* 101:143e51.

28 Brown, A. and Harries, V. (2015), "Infant Sleep and Night Feeding Patterns During Later Infancy: Association with Breastfeeding Frequency, Daytime Complementary Food Intake, and Infant Weight," *Breastfeeding Medicine*, 10(5), 246–252. https://doi.org/10.1089/bfm.2014.0153; Rudzik, A. E. F. and Ball, H. L. (2016), "Exploring maternal perceptions of infant sleep and feeding method among mothers in the United Kingdom: a qualitative focus group study," *Maternal and Child Health Journal*, 20: 33e40.

29 Tikotzky L., Sadeh A., Volkovich E. et al. (2015), "Infant sleep development from 3 to 6 months postpartum: links with maternal sleep and paternal involvement," *Monographs of the Society for Research in Child Development*, 80: 107e24.

30 Pilyoung K., Feldman R., Mayes, L. C. et al. (2011), "Breastfeeding, brain activation to own infant cry, and maternal sensitivity," *Journal of Child Psychology and Psychiatry*, 52: 907e15.

31 Brown, A. and Harries, V. (2015), "Infant Sleep and Night Feeding Patterns During Later Infancy: Association with Breastfeeding Frequency, Daytime Complementary Food Intake, and Infant Weight," *Breastfeeding Medicine*, 10(5) DOI: 10.1089/bfm.2014.0153.

32 Madar, A. A., Kurniasari, A., Marjerrison, N., and Mdala, I. (2024), "Breastfeeding and Sleeping Patterns Among 6–12-Month-Old Infants in Norway," *Maternal and Child Health Journal*, 28(3), 496–505. https://doi.org/10.1007/s10995-023-03805-2.

6. A bed of one's own?

1 In addition to the homemade crib in the spare bedroom, we also had a travel crib in the living room where I was able to park my daughter during the day.

2 Davies, P. (1994), "Ethnicity & SIDS: What have we learnt?," *Early Human Development*, 38: 215–220S.

3 For a thorough systematic review of the research and discourse around this topic, see Mileva-Seitz, V. R., Bakermans-Kranenburg, M. J., Battaini, C., and Luijk, M. P. C. M. (2017), "Parent-child bed-sharing: The good, the bad, and the burden of evidence," *Sleep Medicine Reviews*, 32, 4–27. https://doi.org/10.1016/j.smrv.2016.03.003.

4 Small, M. (1992), "A Reasonable Sleep," *Discover*, April, 83–88.

5 McKenna, J. J., Mosko, S. S., and Richard, C. A. (1997), "Bedsharing promotes breastfeeding," *Pediatrics*, 100(2 Pt 1), 214–219.

6 Mosko, S., Richard, C., McKenna, J., and Drummond, S. (1996), "Infant sleep architecture during bedsharing and possible implications for SIDS," *Sleep*, 19(9), 677–684; Mosko, S., Richard, C., and McKenna, J. (1997), "Maternal sleep and arousals during bedsharing with infants" *Sleep*, 20(2), 142–150; Mosko, S., Richard, C., and McKenna, J. J. (1997), "Infant Arousals During Mother-Infant Bed Sharing: Implications for Infant Sleep and Sudden Infant Death Syndrome Research," *Pediatrics*, 100(5), 841–849. https://doi.org/10.1542/peds.100.5.841.

7 McKenna, J. J., Ball, H. L., and Gettler, L. T. (2007), "Mother–infant cosleeping, breastfeeding and sudden infant death syndrome: What biological anthropology has discovered about normal infant sleep and pediatric sleep medicine," *American Journal of Physical Anthropology,* 134(S45), 133–161; McKenna, J. J. and Gettler, L. T. (2016), "There is no such thing as infant sleep, there is no such thing as breastfeeding, there is only breastsleeping," *Acta Paediatrica*, 105(1), 17–21. https://doi.org/10.1111/apa.13161.

8 Young, J., Fleming, P., Blair, P., and Pollard, K. (2001), "Night-time infant care practices: A longitudinal study of the importance of close contact between mothers and their babies," *Stillmanagement Und Laktation* [Breastfeeding and Lactation Management], 4, 179–210.

9 Fleming, P. J., Young, J., and Blair, P. S. (2006), "The importance of mother-baby interactions in determining night time

thermal conditions for sleeping infants: Observations from the home and sleep laboratory," *Paediatrics and Child Health*, 11(5 Supplement May–June), 7A–11A.

10 Ball, H. L., Hooker, E., and Kelly, P. J. (1999), "Where Will the Baby Sleep? Attitudes and Practices of New and Experienced Parents Regarding Cosleeping with Their Newborn Infants," *American Anthropologist*, 101(1), 143–151. https://doi.org/10.1525/aa.1999.101.1.143.

11 Ball, H. L. (2002), "Reasons to bed-share: Why parents sleep with their infants," *Journal of Reproductive and Infant Psychology*, 20(4), 207–221. https://doi.org/10.1080/0264683021000033147; Ball, H. L. (2003), "Breastfeeding, Bed-Sharing, and Infant Sleep," *Birth*, 30(3), 181–188. https://doi.org/10.1046/j.1523-536X.2003.00243.x.

12 Ball, H. L. (2002), "Reasons to bed-share: Why parents sleep with their infants," *Journal of Reproductive and Infant Psychology*, 20(4), 207–221. https://doi.org/10.1080/0264683021000033147.

13 Confidential Enquiry into Sudden Death in Infancy.

14 Blair, P. S. and Ball, H. L. (2004), "The prevalence and characteristics associated with parent-infant bed-sharing in England," *Archives of Disease in Childhood*, 89(12), 1106–1110. https://doi.org/10.1136/adc.2003.038067.

15 Tuohy, P. G., Smale, P., and Clements, M. (1998), "Ethnic differences in parent/infant co-sleeping practices in New Zealand," *The New Zealand Medical Journal*, 111(1074), 364–366; Gibson, E., Dembofsky, C. A., Rubin, S., and Greenspan, J. S. (2000), "Infant Sleep Position Practices 2 Years Into the 'Back to Sleep' Campaign," *Clinical Pediatrics*, 39(5), 285–289; Rigda, R. S., McMillen, I. C., and Buckley, P. (2000), "Bed sharing patterns in a cohort of Australian infants during the first six months after birth," *Journal of Paediatrics and Child Health*, 36(2), 117–121; Ball, H. L. (2002), "Reasons to bed-share: Why parents sleep with their infants," *Journal of Reproductive and Infant Psychology*, 20(4), 207–221; Brenner, R. A., Simons-Morton,

B. G., Bhaskar, B., Revenis, M., Das, A., and Clemens, J. D. (2003), "Infant-parent bed sharing in an inner-city population," *Archives of Pediatrics & Adolescent Medicine*, 157(1), 33–39; Willinger, M., Ko, C., and Hoffman, H. (2003), "Trends in infant bed sharing in the United States, 1993–2000: the National Infant Sleep Position study," *Archives of Pediatrics*, 157, 43–49; Van Sleuwen, B. (2003), "Infant care practices related to cot death in Turkish and Moroccan families in the Netherlands," *Archives of Disease in Childhood*, 88(9), 784–788; Blair, P. S. and Ball, H. L. (2004), "The prevalence and characteristics associated with parent-infant bed-sharing in England," *Archives of Disease in Childhood*, 89(12), 1106–1110; Bolling, K., Grant, C., Hamlyn, B., and Thornton, A. (2007), "*Infant feeding survey 2005*," London: The Information Centre for Health and Social Care; Hauck, F. R., Signore, C., Fein, S. B., and Raju, T. N. K. (2008), "Infant sleeping arrangements and practices during the first year of life," *Pediatrics*, *122* (Supplement 2), S113. https://doi.org/10.1542/peds.2008-13150; Ateah, C. A. and Hamelin, K. J. (2008), "Maternal bed-sharing practices, experiences, and awareness of risks," *Journal of Obstetric, Gynecologic, and Neonatal Nursing: JOGNN / NAACOG*, 37(3), 274–281.

16 Tomori, C. (2014), *Nighttime Breastfeeding. An American Cultural Dilemma*. Berghahn; Salm Ward, T. C. (2015), "Reasons for mother-infant bed-sharing: a systematic narrative synthesis of the literature and implications for future research," *Maternal and Child Health Journal*, 19(3), 675–690. https://doi.org/10.1007/s10995-014-1557-1.

17 A hazardous arrangement as the baby does not have clear space; we made sure this family received a safe space for their baby when we discovered their sleeping arrangements.

18 Barry, E. S. and McKenna, J. J. (2022), "Reasons mothers bed-share: A review of its effects on infant behavior and development," *Infant Behavior and Development*, 66. https://doi.org/10.1016/j.infbeh.2021.101684.

19 "MacGyvered" references the eighties U.S. TV show *MacGyver* where the lead character would engineer vital equipment from common everyday items.

20 Baddock, S. A., Galland, B. C., Taylor, B. J., and Bolton, D. P. G. (2007), "Sleep arrangements and behavior of bed-sharing families in the home setting," *Pediatrics*, 119(1), e200-7. https://doi.org/10.1542/peds.2006-0744.

21 Ball, H. L., Ward-Platt, M. P., Heslop, E., Leech, S. J., and Brown, K. A. (2006), "Randomised trial of infant sleep location on the postnatal ward," *Archives of Disease in Childhood*, 91(12), 1005–1010. https://doi.org/10.1136/adc.2006.099416.

22 Marinelli, K. A., Ball, H. L., McKenna, J. J., and Blair, P. S. (2019), "An Integrated Analysis of Maternal-Infant Sleep, Breastfeeding, and Sudden Infant Death Syndrome Research Supporting a Balanced Discourse," *Journal of Human Lactation*, 35(3), 510–520. https://doi.org/10.1177/0890334419851797.

23 Ball, H. L. (2006), "Parent-Infant Bedsharing Behavior: Effects of Feeding Type and Presence of Father," *Human Nature*, 17(3), 301–318.

24 Small, M. F. (1998), *Our Babies Ourselves: How Biology and Culture Shape the Way We Parent*. New York: Doubleday Dell Publishing Group.

25 World Health Organization. *Implementation guidance: protecting, promoting and supporting breastfeeding in facilities providing maternity and newborn services—the revised Baby-friendly Hospital Initiative*. Geneva; 2018. Report No.: CC BY-NC-SA 3.0 IGO.

26 Dumas L. (2021), "Remembering Dr. Ann-Marie Widström," *J. Hum. Lact.*, May, 37(2):236. doi: 10.1177/08903344219951 27.

27 Brimdyr, K., Cadwell, K., Svensson, K., Takahashi, Y., Nissen, E., Widström, A. M. (2020), "The nine stages of skin-to-skin: practical guidelines and insights from four countries," *Maternal & Child Nutrition*, October, 16(4): e13042. doi: 10.1111/mcn.13042.

28 Yamauchi, Y. and Yamanouchi, I. (1990), "The Relationship between Rooming-in/not Rooming-in and Breast-Feeding Variables," *Acta*

Paediatrica, 79(11), 1017–1022. https://doi.org/10.1111/j.1651-2227.1990.tb11377.x; Buxton, K. E., Gielen, A. C., Faden, R. R., Brown, C. H., Paige, D. M., and Chwalow, A. J. (1991), "Women intending to breastfeed: predictors of early infant feeding experiences," *American Journal of Preventive Medicine*, 7(2), 101–106.

29 Waldenström, U. and Swenson, Å. (1991), "Rooming-in at night in the postpartum ward," *Midwifery*, 7(2), 82–89. https://doi.org/10.1016/S0266-6138(05)80232-3; Keefe, M. R. (1988), "The Impact of Infant Rooming-In on Maternal Sleep at Night," *Journal of Obstetric, Gynecologic & Neonatal Nursing*, 17(2), 122–126. https://doi.org/10.1111/j.1552-6909.1988.tb00522.x.

30 Ball, H. L., Ward-Platt, M. P., Heslop, E., Leech, S. J., and Brown, K. A. (2006), "Randomised trial of infant sleep location on the postnatal ward," *Archives of Disease in Childhood*, 91(12), 1005–1010. https://doi.org/10.1136/adc.2006.099416.

31 Tennekoon, K. H., Arulambalam, P. D., Karunanayake, E. H., and Seneviratne, H. R. (1994), "Prolactin response to suckling in a group of fully breastfeeding women during the early postpartum period," *Asia Oceania Journal of Obstetrics and Gynaecology*, 20(3), 311–319.

32 Neville, M. C., Morton, J., and Umemura, S. (2001), "Lactogenesis. The transition from pregnancy to lactation," *Pediatric Clinics of North America*, 48, 35–52; Chapman, D. J. and Perez-Escamilla, R. (1999), "Identification of risk factors for delayed onset of lactation," *Journal of the American Dietetic Association*, 99(4), 450–454.

33 Riordan, J. and Auerbach, K. G. (eds.) (1993), *Breastfeeding and Human Lactation*. Boston, MA: Jones and Bartlett. Marasco, L. and Barger, J. (1999), "Cue feeding: Wisdom and science," *Breastfeeding Abstracts*, 18(4), 28–29; Lawrence, R. A. and Lawrence, R. M. (1999), *Breastfeeding: A Guide for the Medical Profession*. Mosby.

34 Gatti, L. (2008), "Maternal Perceptions of Insufficient Milk Supply in Breastfeeding," *Journal of Nursing Scholarship*, 40:

355–363. https://doi.org/10.1111/j.1547-5069.2008.00234.x; Segura-Pérez, S., Richter, L., Rhodes, E. C., Hromi-Fiedler, A., Vilar-Compte, M., Adnew, M., Nyhan, K., and Pérez-Escamilla, R. (2022), "Risk factors for self-reported insufficient milk during the first 6 months of life: A systematic review," *Maternal & Child Nutrition*, 18(S3): e13353. https://doi.org/10.1111/mcn.13353.

35 Ball, H. L., Ward-Platt, M. P., Howel, D., and Russell, C. (2011), "Randomised trial of sidecar crib use on breastfeeding duration (NECOT)," *Archives of Disease in Childhood*, 96(7), 630–634. https://doi.org/10.1136/adc.2010.205344.

36 Robinson, L. (2014), *The impact of mother-infant postnatal proximity and birth intervention on breastfeeding outcomes.* PhD thesis. Durham University.

37 Tully, K. P. and Ball, H. L. (2012), "Postnatal Unit Bassinet Types When Rooming-In after Cesarean Birth: Implications for Breastfeeding and Infant Safety," *Journal of Human Lactation*, 28, 495–505. https://doi.org/10.1177/0890334412452932.

38 Tully, K. P. and Ball, H. L. (2018), "Understanding and enabling breastfeeding in the context of maternal-infant needs" in Tomori, C., Palmquist, A. E. L., and Quinn, E. (eds.), *Breastfeeding: New Anthropological Approaches*, pp. 199–211. Routledge.

39 Howel, D. and Ball, H. L. (2013), "Association between length of exclusive breastfeeding and subsequent breastfeeding continuation," *Journal of Human Lactation*, 29(4), 579–585. https://doi.org/10.1177/0890334413492908.

40 Ball, H. L., Howel, D., Bryant, A., Best, E., Russell, C., and Ward-Platt, M. (2016), "Bed-sharing by breastfeeding mothers: who bed-shares and what is the relationship with breastfeeding duration?," *Acta Paediatrica*, 105(6), 628–634. https://doi.org/10.1111/apa.13354.

41 Tully, K. P. and Ball, H. L. (2013), "Trade-offs underlying maternal breastfeeding decisions: a conceptual model," *Maternal & Child Nutrition*, 9(1), 90–98. https://doi.org/10.1111/j.1740-8709.2011.00378.x.

42 Ball, H. L. (2003), "Breastfeeding, Bed-Sharing, and Infant Sleep," *Birth*, 30(3), 181–188. https://doi.org/10.1046/j.1523-536X.2003.00243.x.

43 McKenna, J. J. and Gettler, L. T. (2016), "There is no such thing as infant sleep, there is no such thing as breastfeeding, there is only breastsleeping," *Acta Paediatrica*, 105(1), 17–21. https://doi.org/10.1111/apa.13161.

44 Hamlyn, B., Brooker, S., Oleinikova, K. and Wands, S. (2002), *Infant Feeding 2000*. The Stationery Office, London.

45 Blair, P. S., Ball, H. L., Pease, A., and Fleming, P. J. (2023), "Bed-sharing and SIDS: an evidence-based approach," *Archives of Disease in Childhood*, 108(4), e6–e6. https://doi.org/10.1136/archdischild-2021-323469.

46 Gettler, L. T., McKenna, J. J., McDade, T. W., Agustin, S. S., and Kuzawa, C. W. (2012), "Does cosleeping contribute to lower testosterone levels in fathers? Evidence from the Philippines," *PLOS ONE*, 7(9), e41559. https://doi.org/10.1371/journal.pone.0041559; Gettler, L. T., Kuo, P. X., Sarma, M. S., Lefever, J. E. B., Cummings, E. M., McKenna, J. J., and Braungart-Rieker, J. M. (2021), "U.S. fathers' reports of bonding, infant temperament and psychosocial stress based on family sleep arrangements," *Evolution, Medicine, and Public Health*, 9(1), 460–469. https://doi.org/10.1093/emph/eoab038.

7. Do not go gentle into that good night

1 https://www.statista.com/statistics/281501/infant-mortality-rate-in-the-united-kingdom/#statisticContainer.

2 While SUDI rates have continued to gradually decline in the UK over the last 30 years, in the U.S. there has been little to no decrease in infant sleep-related deaths since 1994, despite aggressive public health campaigns (Salm Ward, 2020).

3 Kennedy, B. (2016), *Sudden Unexpected Death in Infancy and Childhood: Multi-agency Guidelines for Care and Investigation.* London: The Royal College of Pathologists.

4 Willinger, M., James, L. S., and Catz, C. (1991), "Defining the Sudden Infant Death Syndrome (SIDS): Deliberations of an Expert Panel Convened by the National Institute of Child Health and Human Development," *Pediatric Pathology*, 11(5), 677–684. https://doi.org/10.3109/15513819109065465.

5 Garstang J., Pease, A. S. (2018), "A United Kingdom Perspective," in Duncan, J. R., Byard, R. W. (eds), *SIDS Sudden Infant and Early Childhood Death: The Past, the Present and the Future*, Chapter 18. Adelaide (AU): University of Adelaide Press.

6 https://www.bbc.co.uk/news/uk-england-oxfordshire-64134208.

7 This is the focus of our most recent work. See Ball, H. L. et al. (2024), "Piloting Eyes on the Baby: A Multiagency Training and Implementation Intervention Linking Sudden Unexpected Infant Death Prevention and Safeguarding," *Health & Social Care in the Community.* https://doi.org/10.1155/2024/4944268.

8 Bartick, M. and Tomori, C. (2019), "Sudden infant death and social justice: A syndemics approach," *Maternal & Child Nutrition*, 15(1). https://doi.org/10.1111/mcn.12652.

9 Harrison, L. (2022), *Losing Sleep.* New York University Press. This book is highly recommended for anyone interested in the negative consequences of poorly designed public health interventions.

10 Cowgill, B. (2018), *Rest Uneasy: Sudden Infant Death Syndrome in Twentieth-Century America.* Rutgers University Press.

11 Gilbert, R., Salanti, G., Harden, M., and See, S. (2005), "Infant sleeping position and the sudden infant death syndrome: Systematic review of observational studies and historical review of recommendations from 1940 to 2002," *International Journal of Epidemiology*, 34(4), 874–887. https://doi.org/10.1093/ije/dyi088.

12 Hackett, M. (2012), *Back to Sleep: Creation, Conflict and Consequences of a Public Health Campaign*. Akademiker Verlag.

13 Horne, R. S. C. (2020), "How Pathophysiology Explains Risk and Protective Factors," in Moon, R. (eds.), *Infant Safe Sleep*. Springer, Cham. https://doi.org/10.1007/978-3-030-47542-0_2.

14 Hunt, C. E., Lesko, S. M., Vezina, R. M., McCoy, R., Corwin, M. J., Mandell, F., Willinger, M., Hoffman, H. J., and Mitchell, A. A. (2003), "Infant Sleep Position and Associated Health Outcomes," *Archives of Pediatrics & Adolescent Medicine*, 157(5), 469. https://doi.org/10.1001/archpedi.157.5.469.

15 Gilbert, R., Salanti, G., Harden, M., and See, S. (2005), "Infant sleeping position and the sudden infant death syndrome: Systematic review of observational studies and historical review of recommendations from 1940 to 2002," *International Journal of Epidemiology*, 34(4), 874–887. https://doi.org/10.1093/ije/dyi088.

16 Blair, P. S., Fleming, P. J., Smith, I. J., Platt, M. W., Young, J., Nadin, P., Berry, P. J., and Golding, J., "Babies sleeping with parents: case-control study of factors influencing the risk of the sudden infant death syndrome," *BMJ*. 1999 319(7223): 1457–61. doi: 10.1136/bmj.319.7223.1457; Carpenter, R. G., Irgens, L. M., Blair, P. S., England, P. D., Fleming, P., Huber, J., et al. (2004), "Sudden unexplained infant death in 20 regions in Europe: case control study," *Lancet*, 363(9404): 185-91; Blair, P. S., Platt, M. W., Smith, I. J., and Fleming, P. J., "Sudden Infant Death Syndrome and the time of death: factors associated with night-time and day-time deaths," *International Journal of Epidemiology*, 2006; 35(6): 1563–9. doi: 10.1093/ije/dyl212.

17 Horne, R. S. C. (2020), "How Pathophysiology Explains Risk and Protective Factors," in Moon, R. (ed.), *Infant Safe Sleep*. Springer, Cham. https://doi.org/10.1007/978-3-030-47542-0_2.

18 McKenna, J. J. (1986), "An anthropological perspective on the sudden infant death syndrome (SIDS): the role of parental

breathing cues and speech breathing adaptations.," *Medical Anthropology*, 10(1), 9–92. doi: 10.1080/01459740.1986.9965947; Konner, M. and Super, C. (1987), "Sudden infant death syndrome: An anthropological hypothesis," in Super, C. M. (ed.), *The Role of Culture in Developmental Disorder*, pp. 95–108. Academic Press; McKenna, J. J. et al. (1990), "Sleep and arousal patterns of co-sleeping human mother/infant pairs: a preliminary physiological study with implications for the study of sudden infant death syndrome (SIDS)," *American Journal of Physical Anthropology*, 83(3), 331–47. doi: 10.1002/ajpa.1330830307; Trevathan, W. R., McKenna, J. J. (1994), "Evolutionary environments of human birth and infancy: Insights to apply to contemporary life," *Child. Environ.* 11, 88–104.

19 Salm Ward, T. C. (2020), "Safe sleep recommendations," in Moon, R. Y. (ed.), *Infant Safe Sleep: A Pocket Guide for Clinicians,* pp. 49–66. Springer Publishing.

20 Renz-Polster, H., Blair, P. S., Ball, H. L., Jenni, O. G., and De Bock, F. (2024), "Evolutionary-Developmental Theory of Sudden Infant Death Syndrome," *Human Nature*, 35(2), 153–196. https://doi.org/10.1007/s12110-024-09474-6.

21 Horne, R. S. C. (2020), "How Pathophysiology Explains Risk and Protective Factors," in Moon, R. Y. (ed.), *Infant Safe Sleep*. Springer, Cham. https://doi.org/10.1007/978-3-030-47542-0_2.

22 Horne, R. S. C., Franco, P., Adamson, T. M., Groswasser, J., and Kahn, A. (2004), "Influences of maternal cigarette smoking on infant arousability," *Early Human Development*, 79(1), 49–58. https://doi.org/10.1016/j.earlhumdev.2004.04.00.

23 Horne, R. S. C. (2020), "How Pathophysiology Explains Risk and Protective Factors," in Moon, R. Y. (ed.), *Infant Safe Sleep*. Springer, Cham. https://doi.org/10.1007/978-3-030-47542-0_2.

24 Thompson, J. M. D., Tanabe, K., Moon, R. Y., Mitchell, E. A., McGarvey, C., Tappin, D., Blair, P. S., and Hauck, F. R. (2017), "Duration of Breastfeeding and Risk of SIDS: An Individual Par-

ticipant Data Meta-analysis," *Pediatrics*, 140(5), e20171324. https://doi.org/10.1542/peds.2017-1324.

25 Horne, R. S. C., Parslow, P. M., Ferens, D., Watts, A.-M., and Adamson, T. M. (2004), "Comparison of evoked arousability in breast and formula fed infants," *Archives of Disease in Childhood*, 89(1), 22–25; Elias, M. F., Nicolson, N. A., Bora, C., Johnston, J., Elias, F., and Nicolson, A. (1986), "Sleep / Wake Patterns of Breast-Fed Infants in the First 2 Years of Life," *Pediatrics*, 77, 322–329.

26 Dunford, E. K., Popkin, B. M. (2023), "Ultra-processed food for infants and toddlers; dynamics of supply and demand," *Bulletin of the World Health Organization*, May 1; 101(5): 358–360. doi: 10.2471/BLT.22.289448.

27 Salm Ward, T. C. (2020), "Safe sleep recommendations," in Moon, R. Y. (ed.), *Infant Safe Sleep: A Pocket Guide for Clinicians*, pp. 49–66. Springer Publishing.

28 Horne, R. S. C. (2020), "How Pathophysiology Explains Risk and Protective Factors," in Moon, R. Y. (ed.), *Infant Safe Sleep*. Springer, Cham. https://doi.org/10.1007/978-3-030-47542-0_2.

29 Ball, H. L. (2006), "Caring for twin infants: sleeping arrangements and their implications," *Evidence Based Midwifery*, 4(1): 10–16.

30 Ball, H. L. (2007), "Together or apart? A behavioural and physiological investigation of sleeping arrangements for twin babies," *Midwifery*, 23(4), 404–412. https://doi.org/10.1016/j.midw.2006.07.004.

31 Feldman-Winter, L. and Goldsmith, J. P., "Committee on Fetus And Newborn, Task Force on Sudden Infant Death Syndrome; Safe Sleep and Skin-to-Skin Care in the Neonatal Period for Healthy Term Newborns," *Pediatrics* 2016, e20161889. 10.1542/peds.2016-1889.

32 Volpe, L. E. (2010), *Using Life-History Theory to Evaluate the Nighttime Parenting Strategies of First-Time Adolescent and Adult Mothers*. http://etheses.dur.ac.uk/287/.

33 Volpe, L. E., Ball, H. L., and McKenna, J. J. (2013), "Nighttime parenting strategies and sleep-related risks to infants," *Social Science &*

Medicine 79(1), 92–100. https://doi.org/10.1016/j.socscimed.2012.05.043; Volpe, L. E. and Ball, H. L. (2015), "Infant sleep-related deaths: why do parents take risks?," *Archives of Disease in Childhood*, 100(7), 603–604. https://doi.org/10.1136/archdischild-2014-307745.

34 Filiano, J. J. and Kinney, H. C. (1994), "A perspective on neuropathologic findings in victims of the sudden infant death syndrome: the triple-risk model," *Neonatology*, 65, pp. 194–197. doi: 10.1159/000244052.

35 Filiano, J. J. and Kinney, H. C. (1994), "A perspective on neuropathologic findings in victims of the sudden infant death syndrome: the triple-risk model," *Neonatology*, 65, pp. 194–197. doi: 10.1159/000244052.

36 Renz-Polster, H., Blair, P. S., Ball, H. L., Jenni, O. G., and de Bock, F. (2024), "Death from Failed Protection? An Evolutionary-Developmental Theory of Sudden Infant Death Syndrome," *Human Nature*, 35(2), 153–196. https://doi.org/10.1007/s12110-024-09474-6.

37 As noted in Chapter 6, in this book co-sleeping covers all situations where adult(s) and infant(s) sleep together on the same surface, while bed-sharing is a subset of co-sleeping that specifically refers to adult(s) and infant(s) sleeping on an adult bed. McKenna's definition of co-sleeping as any shared sleep environment (e.g., encompassing room-sharing) is not used here due to its breadth and the need to distinguish between sleep surfaces.

38 Ball, H. L. (2017), "The Atlantic Divide: Contrasting U.K. and U. S. Recommendations on Cosleeping and Bed-Sharing," *Journal of Human Lactation*, 33(4), 765–769. https://doi.org/10.1177/0890334417713943; Salm Ward, T. C. (2020), "Safe sleep recommendations," in Moon, R. Y. (ed.), *Infant Safe Sleep: A Pocket Guide for Clinicians*, pp. 49–66. Springer Publishing.

39 https://www.nice.org.uk/guidance/ng194/evidence/n-cosleeping-risk-factors-pdf-326764485978.

40 https://www.ncmd.info/wp-content/uploads/2022/12/SUDIC-Thematic-report_FINAL.pdf.

41 Blair, P. S., Sidebotham, P., Pease, A., and Fleming, P. J. (2014), "Bed-Sharing in the Absence of Hazardous Circumstances: Is There a Risk of Sudden Infant Death Syndrome? An Analysis from Two Case-Control Studies Conducted in the UK," *PLOS ONE*, 9(9), e107799. https://doi.org/10.1371/journal.pone.0107799.

42 https://www.nice.org.uk/guidance/qs37/chapter/Quality-statement-5-Safer-practices-for-bed-sharing.

43 In addition to the UK, risk minimization is used in parts of Europe (e.g., Spain, Norway), some Australian states (e.g., Queensland) and Canadian provinces (e.g., British Columbia) and probably other places too.

44 Carpenter, R., McGarvey, C., Mitchell, E. A, Tappin, D. M., Vennemann, M. M., Smuk, M., and Carpenter, J. R. (2013), "Bed sharing when parents do not smoke: is there a risk of SIDS? An individual level analysis of five major case–control studies," *BMJ Open*, 3(5), e002299. https://doi.org/10.1136/bmjopen-2012-002299.

45 https://borninbradford.nhs.uk.

46 Ball, H. L. et al. (2012), "Infant care practices related to sudden infant death syndrome in South Asian and White British families in the UK," *Paediatric and Perinatal Epidemiology*, 26(1), pp. 3–12. doi: 10.1111/j.1365-3016.2011.01217.x; Ball, H. L. et al. (2012), "Bed- and Sofa-Sharing Practices in a UK Biethnic Population," *Pediatrics*, 129(3), pp. e673–e681. doi: 10.1542/peds.2011-1964.

47 Crane, D. and Ball, H. L. (2016), "A qualitative study in parental perceptions and understanding of SIDS-reduction guidance in a UK bi-cultural urban community," *BMC Pediatrics*, 16(1), p. 23. doi: 10.1186/s12887-016-0560-7.

48 Bamber, A. R., Pryce, J., Ashworth, M. T. et al. (2014), "Sudden unexpected infant deaths associated with car seats," *Forensic Science,*

Medicine and Pathology, 10, 187–192. https://doi.org/10.1007/s12024-013-9524-5; Liaw, P., Moon, R. Y., Han, A., and Colvin, J. D. (2019), "Infant Deaths in Sitting Devices," *Pediatrics*, 144 (1): e20182576.10.1542/peds.2018-2576.

49 Righard, L. and Alade, M. (1997), "Breastfeeding and the use of pacifiers," *Birth*, 24(2): 116–20; Victora, C. et al. (1997), "Pacifier use and short breastfeeding duration. Cause, Consequence or Coincidence," *Pediatrics*, 99(3): 445–453.

50 Blair, P. S. and Fleming, P. J. (2006), "Dummies and SIDS: Causality has not been established," *BMJ*, 332: 178.

51 Pease, A. S., Fleming, P. J., Hauck, F. R., Moon, R. Y., Horne, R. S., L'Hoir, M. P., Ponsonby, A. L., and Blair, P. S. (2016), "Swaddling and the Risk of Sudden Infant Death Syndrome: A Meta-analysis," *Pediatrics*, June, 137(6): e20153275. doi: 10.1542/peds.2015-3275.

52 Dixley, A. and Ball, H. L. (2023), "The impact of swaddling upon breastfeeding: A critical review," *American Journal of Human Biology*. doi: 10.1002/ajhb.23878; Dixley, A. and Ball, H. L. (2022), "The effect of swaddling on infant sleep and arousal: A systematic review and narrative synthesis," *Frontiers in Pediatrics*. doi: 10.3389/fped.2022.1000180.

53 https://www.lullabytrust.org.uk/wp-content/uploads/The-Lullaby-Trust-Product-Guide-Web.pdf.

8. The darkest nights

1 Trivers, R. (1972), "Parental investment and sexual selection. Sexual Selection & the Descent of Man," pp. 136–179. Aldine de Gruyter, New York; Trivers, R. (1974), "Parent-Offspring Conflict," *American Zoologist*, 14 (1): 249–264.

2 Blurton Jones, N. G. and Costa, E. da. (1987), "A suggested adaptive value of toddler night waking: Delaying the birth of the

next sibling," *Ethology and Sociobiology*, 8(2), 135–142. https://doi.org/10.1016/0162-3095(87)90036-7.

3 Ball, H. L. and Panter-Brick, C. (2001), "Child survival and the modulation of parental investment" in Ellison, P. (ed.), *Reproductive ecology and human evolution*, pp. 249–266. Aldine de Gruyter.

4 Hrdy, S. B. (2001), *Mother Nature: A History of Mothers, Nature and Natural Selection*. Pantheon.

5 Hrdy, S. B. (2024), *Father Time: A Natural History of Men and Babies*. Princeton University Press.

6 Haig, D. (2014), "Troubled sleep: Night waking, breastfeeding and parent-offspring conflict," *Evolution, Medicine, and Public Health*, 32–39. https://doi.org/10.1093/emph/eou005.

7 Ou, C. H., Hall, W. A., Rodney, P., and Stremler, R. (2022), "Correlates of Canadian mothers' anger during the postpartum period: a cross-sectional survey," *BMC Pregnancy and Childbirth*, 22(1). https://doi.org/10.1186/s12884-022-04479-4.

8 Teti, D. M., Fronberg, K. M., Fanton, H., and Crosby, B. (2022), "Infant sleep arrangements, infant-parent sleep, and parenting during the first six months post-partum," *Infant Behavior and Development*, 69, 101756.

9 Ekirch, A. R. (2006), *At Day's Close: Night in Time Past*. W. W. Norton & Co.; Samson, D. R. (2021), "The Human Sleep Paradox: The Unexpected Sleeping Habits of *Homo sapiens*," *Annual Review of Anthropology*, 50, 259–274. https://doi.org/10.1146/annurev-anthro-010220-075523.

10 Foster, R. (2022), *Life Time: The New Science of the Body Clock, and How It Can Revolutionize Your Sleep and Health*. Penguin Random House.

11 Ball, H. L. and Keegan, A. A. (2022), "Digital health tools to support parents with parent-infant sleep and mental well-being," *NPJ Digital Medicine*; "The Truth about sleep trackers," *New York Times*, 29.11.2023.

12 Coo Calcagni, S., Bei, B., Milgrom, J., and Trinder, J. (2012), "The relationship between sleep and mood in first-time and experienced

mothers," *Behavioral Sleep Medicine*, 10(3), 167–179. https://doi.org/10.1080/15402002.2012.668147.

13 For example, the case of Daisy-Mae Burrill. http://www.itv.com/news/2016-10-25/father-found-guilty-of-murdering-baby-daughter-by-throwing-her-in-fit-of-temper-for-crying/ Accessed 26 October 2016.

14 Ball, H. L. (2013), "Supporting parents who are worried about their newborn's sleep," *BMJ*, 346(2013), f2344. https://doi.org/10.1136/bmj.f2344; Ball, H. L. (2016), "Babies don't need sleep coaches—but sometimes their parents do . . ." *The Conversation*. https://theconversation.com/babies-dont-need-sleep-coaches-but-sometimes-their-parents-do-70464.

15 Rudzik, A. E. and Ball, H. L. (2016), "Baby-Lag: Methods for assessing parental tiredness and fatigue," in L. L. Seivert and D. E. Brown (eds), *Biological Measures of Human Experience Across the Lifespan: Making Visible the Invisible* (29–46). Springer Verlag. https://doi.org/10.1007/978-3-319-44103-0_3.

16 Paulson, J. F. and Bazemore, S. (2010), "Prenatal and postpartum depression in fathers and its association with maternal depression," *JAMA*, 303: 1962–9. doi: 10.1001/jama.2010.605; Petersen, I., Peltola, T., Kaski, S., Walters, K. R., and Hardoon, S. (2018), "Depression, depressive symptoms and treatments in women who have recently given birth: UK cohort study," *BMJ Open*, 8: e022152. doi: 10.1136/bmjopen-2018-022152.

17 Rudzik, A. E. and Ball, H. L. (2016), "Baby-Lag: Methods for assessing parental tiredness and fatigue," in L. L. Seivert and D. E. Brown (eds), *Biological Measures of Human Experience Across the Lifespan: Making Visible the Invisible* (29–46). Springer Verlag. https://doi.org/10.1007/978-3-319-44103-0_3.

18 Rudzik, A. E. and Ball, H. L. (2016), "Baby-Lag: Methods for assessing parental tiredness and fatigue," in L. L. Seivert and D. E. Brown (eds), *Biological Measures of Human Experience Across the*

Lifespan: Making Visible the Invisible (29–46). Springer Verlag. https://doi.org/10.1007/978-3-319-44103-0_3.

19 Newland, R. P., Parade, S. H., Fisk, J., Dickstein, S., and Seifer, R. (2016), "Goodness of fit between maternal and infant sleep: Associations with maternal depressive symptoms and attachment security," *Infant Behavior and Development*, 44, 179–188. https://doi.org/10.1016/j.infbeh.2016.06.010; Tikotzky, L. (2016), "Postpartum Maternal Sleep, Maternal Depressive Symptoms and Self-Perceived Mother–Infant Emotional Relationship," *Behavioral Sleep Medicine*, 14(1), 5–22. https://doi.org/10.1080/15402002.2014.940111.

20 Sponsored by Johnson & Johnson, manufacturers of baby bath and bedtime products.

21 Mindell, J. A., Sadeh, A., Wiegand, B., How, T. H., and Goh, D. Y. T. (2010), "Cross-cultural differences in infant and toddler sleep," *Sleep Medicine*, 11(3), 274–280.

22 Gottlieb, A. (2000), "Where have all the babies gone? Toward an Anthropology of Infants (and their Caretakers)," *Anthropological Quarterly*, 73(3), 121–132. https://muse.jhu.edu/article/2062.

23 Crittenden, A. N., Samson, D. R., Herlosky, K. N., Mabulla, I. A., Mabulla, A. Z. P., and McKenna, J. J. (2018), "Infant co-sleeping patterns and maternal sleep quality among Hadza hunter-gatherers," *Sleep Health*, 4(6), 527–534. https://doi.org/10.1016/j.sleh.2018.10.005.

24 https://assets.publishing.service.gov.uk/media/5a7eb7a0ed915d74e33f1fae/SACN_Statement_on_Good-Night_Milks_2008.pdf.

25 https://www.masadaprivate.com.au/Early-Parenting-Centre/Residential-Program.

26 https://www.newyorker.com/magazine/2021/06/28/the-promise-and-the-peril-of-a-high-priced-sleep-trainer.

27 St. James-Roberts, I., Sleep, J., Morris, S., Owen, C., and Gillham, P. (2001), "Use of a behavioural programme in the first 3 months to prevent infant crying and sleeping problems,"

Journal of Paediatrics and Child Health, 37(3), 289–297. https://doi.org/10.1046/j.1440-1754.2001.00699.x.

28 Paul, I. M., Savage, J. S., Anzman-Frasca, S., Marini, M. E., Mindell, J. A., and Birch, L. L. (2016), "INSIGHT Responsive Parenting Intervention and Infant Sleep," *Pediatrics*, 138(1), e20160762–e20160762. https://doi.org/10.1542/peds.2016-0762.

29 Matthew Aney, "Babywise" advice linked to dehydration, failure to thrive. *AAP News,* April 1998, 14 (4): 21. 10.1542/14.4.21.

30 Gordon, M. (2023), "Parental experiences with the promise of extinction," Symposium Presentation World Infant Mental Health Conference, Dublin, Ireland.

31 Skinner B. F. (1984), "The evolution of behaviour," *Journal of the Experimental Analysis of Behavior*, 41: 217–21.

32 Etherton, H., Blunden, S., and Hauck, Y., "Discussion of extinction-based behavioral sleep interventions for young children and reasons why parents may find them difficult," *Journal of Clinical Sleep Medicine*, 2016; 12(11): 1535–1543.

33 Douglas, P. S. and Hill, P. S. (2013), "Behavioral sleep interventions in the first six months of life do not improve outcomes for mothers or infants: a systematic review," *Journal of Developmental and Behavioral Pediatrics*, 34(7), 497–507. https://doi.org/10.1097/DBP.0b013e31829cafa6.

34 Gerhardt, S. (2004), *Why love matters: how affection shapes a baby's brain.* Routledge.

35 Kempler, L., Sharpe, L., Miller, C. B., and Bartlett, D. J. (2016), "Do psychosocial sleep interventions improve infant sleep or maternal mood in the postnatal period? A systematic review and meta-analysis of randomised controlled trials," *Sleep Medicine Reviews*, 29(1), 15–22. https://doi.org/10.1016/j.smrv.2015.08.002.

36 Gordon, M. (2023), "Why the 'research base' of crying-it-out isn't all it's cracked up to be." https://www.littlelivewires.com/post/research-on-crying-it-out.

37 Loutzenhiser, L., Hoffman, J., and Beatch, J. (2014), "Parental perceptions of the effectiveness of graduated extinction in reducing infant night-wakings." *Journal of Reproductive and Infant Psychology*, 32(3), 282–291.

38 Etherton, H., Blunden, S., and Hauck, Y. (2016), "Discussion of Extinction-Based Behavioral Sleep Interventions for Young Children and Reasons Why Parents May Find Them Difficult," *Journal of Clinical Sleep Medicine*, 12 (11): 1535–1543). https://doi.org/10.5664/jcsm.6284.

39 Review of "Every child can learn to sleep" on Kids Nook http://kids-nook.com/advice/every-child-can-learn-to-sleep/.

40 Blunden, S. and Dawson, D. (2020), "Behavioural sleep interventions in infants: Plan B—Combining models of responsiveness to increase parental choice," *Journal of Paediatrics and Child Health*, 56(5):675-679. doi: 10.1111/jpc.14818.

41 Blunden, S., Osborne, J., and King, Y. (2022), "Do responsive sleep interventions impact mental health in mother/infant dyads compared to extinction interventions? A pilot study," *Archives of Women's Mental Health*, 25(3), 621–631.

42 www.basisonline.org.uk. Launched in April 2012 as the Infant Sleep Info Source (ISIS) it was grudgingly renamed as Baby Sleep Info Source (Basis) in 2018 after hearing too many stories about parents being fearful to type ISIS into their search engine—at which point the terrorist organization commonly known as ISIS promptly disappeared from the nightly news. ISIS/Basis was developed in collaboration with Unicef UK Baby Friendly Initiative, NCT (formerly National Childbirth Trust), and La Leche League GB, with funding from the Economic & Social Research Council. It was later endorsed by the other UK breastfeeding organizations.

43 Galland, B. C., Sayers, R. M., Cameron, S. L., Gray, A. R., Heath, A.-L. M., Lawrence, J. A., Newlands, A., Taylor, B. J., and Taylor, R. W. (2017), "Anticipatory guidance to prevent infant sleep problems

within a randomised controlled trial: infant, maternal and partner outcomes at 6 months of age," *BMJ Open*, 7(5), e014908. https://doi.org/10.1136/bmjopen-2016-014908.

44 Stremler, R., Hodnett, E., Kenton, L., Lee, K., Weiss, S., Weston, J., and Willan, A. (2013), "Effect of behavioural-educational intervention on sleep for primiparous women and their infants in early postpartum: multisite randomised controlled trial," *British Medical Journal*, 346, f1164–f1164. https://doi.org/10.1136/bmj.f1164.

45 Ball, H. L. (2013), "Supporting parents who are worried about their newborn's sleep," *BMJ*, 346(2013), f2344–f2344. https://doi.org/10.1136/bmj.f2344.

46 Galland, B. C., Sayers, R. M., Cameron, S. L., Gray, A. R., Heath, A.-L. M., Lawrence, J. A., Newlands, A., Taylor, B. J., and Taylor, R. W. (2017), "Anticipatory guidance to prevent infant sleep problems within a randomised controlled trial: infant, maternal and partner outcomes at 6 months of age," *BMJ Open*, 7(5), e014908. https://doi.org/10.1136/bmjopen-2016-014908.

47 Santos, I. S., Del-Ponte, B., Tovo-Rodrigues, L., Halal, C. S., Matijasevich, A., Cruz, S., Anselmi, L., Silveira, M. F., Hallal, P. R. C., and Bassani, D. G. (2019), "Effect of Parental Counseling on Infants' Healthy Sleep Habits in Brazil: A Randomized Clinical Trial," *JAMA Network Open*, 2(12), e1918062. https://doi.org/10.1001/jamanetworkopen.2019.18062.

48 Kempler, L., Sharpe, L., Miller, C. B., and Bartlett, D. J. (2016), "Do psychosocial sleep interventions improve infant sleep or maternal mood in the postnatal period? A systematic review and meta-analysis of randomised controlled trials," *Sleep Medicine Reviews*, 29(1), 15–22. https://doi.org/10.1016/j.smrv.2015.08.002.

49 For example, the Beyond Sleep Training Project established by Carly Grubb in Australia in 2017, which now supports thousands of members worldwide. https://thebeyondsleeptrainingproject.com/our-story.

9. The sun also rises

1 Basis was awarded a second place prize for "Outstanding Impact in Society" in the first round of ESRC "Celebrating Impact" awards in 2013, and in 2018 Durham University received the Queen's Anniversary Prize for this work.

2 Lynne Murray and Paul Ramchandani had already made a similar suggestion back in 2007, in a commentary in the *Archives of Disease in Childhood*, that had no doubt influenced my thinking.

3 Giallo, R., Cooklin, A., Dunning, M., and Seymour, M. (2014), "The Efficacy of an Intervention for the Management of Postpartum Fatigue," *Journal of Obstetric, Gynecologic & Neonatal Nursing*, 43(5), 598–613. https://doi.org/10.1111/1552-6909.12489.

4 Whittingham, K. and Douglas, P. (2014), "Optimizing parent-infant sleep from birth to 6 months: a new paradigm," *Infant Mental Health Journal*, 35(6), 614–623. https://doi.org/10.1002/imhj.21455; Whittingham, K. and Douglas, P. S. (2016), "Possums—building contextual behavioural science into an evidence-based approach to parenting support in early life," in Kirkcaldy, B. (ed.), *Psychotherapy in Parenthood and Beyond*, pp. 43–56. Edizioni Minerva Medica.

5 https://www.pameladouglas.com.au/possumsoriginstory.

6 Ball, H. L., Douglas, P. S., Kulasinghe, K., Whittingham, K., and Hill, P. (2018), "The Possums Infant Sleep Program: parents' perspectives on a novel parent-infant sleep intervention in Australia," *Sleep Health*, 4(6), 519–526. https://doi.org/10.1016/j.sleh.2018.08.007.

7 In Australia, where GP practices are run as small businesses compensated via an insurance system, Pam and her colleagues had the luxury of hour-long appointments with their patients. To use the Possums Sleep Program in the UK we needed to transform it into something that registered nurses or midwives could offer during much shorter appointments, and deliver in antenatal and postnatal support groups.

8 Created for us by Chris Lavelle of LDi studios. https://www.ldistudios.com.

9 Pseudonym.

10 Ball, H. L., Taylor, C. E., Thomas, V., and Douglas, P. S. (2020), "Development and evaluation of 'Sleep, Baby & You'—An approach to supporting parental well-being and responsive infant caregiving," *PLOS ONE*, 15(8), e0237240. https://doi.org/10.1371/journal.pone.0237240.

11 Kenkel, W. M., Perkeybile, A. M., and Carter, C. S., "The neurobiological causes and effects of alloparenting," *Developmental Neurobiology*, February 2017, 77(2): 214–232. doi: 10.1002/dneu.22465.

12 In *The Discontented Little Baby Book*, published in 2014, Pam summarizes some of the issues that parents brought to her as a practicing GP, and the ways in which she would advise them.

13 I sometimes get asked by parents if I will send them copies of the *Sleep, Baby & You* booklet so they can use the program; however, it is not designed to be a self-help tool, and we don't make it available on the internet for that reason. SBY is a discussion tool for trained practitioners to use with families in conversation about their challenges and potential solutions, and for those families to use as an aide memoir. The full Possums Sleep Program can be used independently by parents, and details can be found at https://possumssleepprogram.com/.

14 By seeking the help of a trained peer supporter or professional at an infant feeding support group or similar.

15 Douglas, P. S. (2014), *The Discontented Little Baby Book*. University of Queensland Press.

16 Ball, H. L., (2022), "What's really going on when a child is 'over-tired' and how to help them go to sleep?," *The Conversation*, December 6. https://theconversation.com/whats-really-going-on-when-a-child-is-overtired-and-how-to-help-them-go-to-sleep-194784.

17 Douglas, P. S. (2014), *The Discontented Little Baby Book.* University of Queensland Press; Whittingham, K. and Douglas, P. (2014), "Optimizing parent-infant sleep from birth to 6 months: a new paradigm," *Infant Mental Health Journal*, 35(6), 614–623. https://doi.org/10.1002/imhj.21455.

18 Whittingham, K. and Douglas, P. (2014), "Optimizing parent-infant sleep from birth to 6 months: a new paradigm," *Infant Mental Health Journal*, 35(6), 614–623. https://doi.org/10.1002/imhj.21455.

19 Dixley, A. and Ball, H. L. (2022), "The effect of swaddling on infant sleep and arousal: A systematic review and narrative synthesis," *Frontiers in Pediatrics*, 10. https://doi.org/10.3389/fped.2022.1000180; Dixley, A. and Ball, H. L. (2023), "The impact of swaddling upon breastfeeding: A critical review," *American Journal of Human Biology*, 35(6). https://doi.org/10.1002/ajhb.23878.

20 In one of our sleep lab videos we observed a three-month-old baby very effectively alert her sleeping father to her presence by vigorously jabbing all four limbs into his back as he leaned toward her, causing him to immediately jump up off the bed.

21 T.I.C.K.S. Rules for Safe Babywearing from the UK Sling Consortium. https://babyslingsafety.co.uk.

Index